Live Longer,
Live Healthier:
The Secrets for Graceful Aging
First Edition

Live Longer, Live Healthier:
The Secrets for Graceful Aging
First Edition

 Midwest Cardiovascular
Research Foundation

Copyright © 2007
Midwest Cardiovascular Research Foundation
1622 E Lombard Street
Davenport, Iowa 52803
Phone: 563-324-2828
Fax: 563-324-2835
www.mcrfmd.com

Library of Congress Control Number: 2007925490
ISBN-13 9780975538425
ISBN-10 0-9755384-2-x

The reader is urged to review the package information data of the manufacturers of any products mentioned.

Printed in the United States of America

Midwest Cardiovascular Research Foundation
1622 E Lombard Street
Davenport, Iowa 52803
Phone: 563-324-2828
Fax: 563-324-2835
www.mcrfmd.com

Illustrator and Graphic Designer: Lynne Majetic, RN, BA
Editors: Suzanne M. Hartung and Jan J. Harper

Live Longer, Live Healthier:
The Secrets for Graceful Aging
First Edition

Nicolas W. Shammas, MD, MS, FACC, FACP
with contributing authors

Illustrator and Graphic Designer:
Lynne Majetic, RN, BA
Editors: Suzanne M. Hartung and Jan J. Harper

Midwest Cardiovascular
Research Foundation

Important Note:
Never Hesitate to Seek Medical Attention!

We hope and intend that this book will help you understand the nature of problems that affect seniors and how to communicate them more effectively with your healthcare provider.

This book – including any and all information, product information, data, text, graphics or other materials that may appear herein – is intended solely for general education and information purposes and is not intended to be used to make medical or health-related decisions without the involvement of healthcare professionals.

The information in this book is not a substitute for, nor does it supersede, professional medical advice.

If you are seeking medical advice, you should consult a physician or other qualified health provider. *Never hesitate to seek medical attention!*

To all the seniors of our community,
including my lovely mother, Vera,
for making this book possible.

To my wonderful family –
my wife, Gail, and our children,
WJ, Andy and Anna,
for their unconditional love, support and
encouragement in editing this book.

Preface xi
Nicolas W. Shammas, MD, MS, FACC, FACP

Chapters

1. **The Epidemiology of an Aging Population** 1
   Jon H. Lemke, PhD, and Amanda K. DeGraeve, BS

2. **Heart Disease as We Grow Older** 13
   Nicolas W. Shammas, MD, MS, FACC, FACP

3. **Peripheral Vascular Disease** 31
   Eric J. Dippel, MD

4. **The Aging Brain** 43
   Rodney A. Short, MD

5. **How to Respond to Emergencies When Every Second Counts** 55
   Lori Christensen, RN

6. **Tips to Reduce High Blood Pressure** 69
   Nidal Harb, MD, FACC, FACP

7. **Diabetes Care: What You Need to Know** 81
   Danita Harrison, ARN, CDE

8. **Osteoporosis: a Leading Cause of Bone Fracture as We Grow Older.** 101
   Susan Freburg, ARNP

9. **Cholesterol, Aging and Heart Disease** 113
   Peter P. Toth, MD, PhD, FAAFP, FCCP, FAHA, FACC

10. **Quitting Smoking: It is Never Too Late** 121
    Chris Pekios, RRT

11. Nutrition as We Age 129
Elaine Guthrie, RD, LD/N

12. The Disease of Obesity 153
Denise Strathdee, LD, LMHC

**13. Stay Active: The Importance of
Exercise as We Age** 169
Karen Doy, MS

**14. Alternative Medicine:
What You Need to Know** 187
John W. Golden, MD

15. What You Need to Know About Cancer 225
*Shobha Chitneni, MD, Sue Clarahan, RD, LD
Karen Crawford, BSN, CRNI, OCN
Faith Damewood, RN, OCN, Stefanie Dreher, RN, OCN
Pam Iverson, RN, OCN*

16. An Overview of Rheumatic Illnesses 241
David B. Staub, MD

17. Erectile Dysfunction and the Golden Age 253
Ghassoub Harb, MD, FACS

**18. Improving Mental Health and Lifestyle as
We Age** 265
Melodee Harris, MSN, APN

**19. Common Orthopedic Problems Encountered as
We Age** 281
*Michael Pyevich, MD, Timothy Milea, MD,
Joseph G. Martin, MD, Steven A. Boardman, MD,
Richard S. Collins, MD*

20. Infections as We Age: How to Recognize the Symptoms and Learn How to Prevent Them 305
Bharat Motwani, MD

21. Eye Diseases of the Elderly. 315
Ashok R. Penmatcha, MD

22. Safe, Graceful Aging – A Plastic Surgeon's Perspective. 337
John M. Searles, Jr., MD, Anne R. Cramer, MD

23. Leaving the Hospital – How to Get the Care You Need 347
Jennifer Busch, LBSW

24. Financial Planning – It's Never Too Late to Start!. 351
J. Clark Arons, FIC, CLU

25. Transportation and Mobility Challenges Faced by Older Drivers. 363
Denise A. Coiner, MS, RTR

26. Research and the Mature Adult 369
Penny Stoakes RN, CCRC

27. How to Talk to Your Doctor! 375
Suzy Hartung, BA

28. How to Engage in Positive, Graceful Living and Aging: Remaining Engaged in Your Community Can Also Enhance Your Own Well-being!. 383
Suzy Hartung, BA

Index. 395

"Growing older is not for wimps," a patient of mine once told me. Despite her share of health problems, she is always joyful, full of life, with a charming smile. "You simply cannot give up! You have to keep the fight and do your best to stay healthy, independent and feel you are always needed," she continued. Listening to my patient turning into my mentor and I her student, the idea of this book came to mind. I realized the need to have an easy-to-read, comprehensive book about "growing older" and staying physically and mentally healthy to enjoy life abundantly and to its fullest.

"Live Longer, Live Healthier: The Secrets for Graceful Aging" is written for a rapidly-growing aging population that intends to "keep the fight." Equipped with the basic knowledge presented in this book, seniors (defined as 55 years of age or older) will have the know-how on how to grow older elegantly and gracefully, staying healthy, independent and socially active. Although heart and blood vessel diseases, cancer, lung diseases, infection and diabetes lead the way in the causes of death as we grow older, there are other issues that need to be addressed, including depression, social isolation, financial problems and so forth. As the aging population grows bigger and lives longer, our socioeconomic system will be faced with new challenges and the role of the elderly in society might need to be redefined.

This book is published by the Midwest Cardiovascular Research Foundation, Davenport, Iowa, established in August of 2002. MCRF is a nonprofit 501(c) (3) public charitable foundation. After the tremendous success of its first book, *"Learn about Your Heart . . . Made Simple"*, the Foundation embarked on the ambitious project of publishing *"Live Longer, Live Healthier: The Secrets for Graceful Aging."* With 26 contributing authors and 28 chapters touching on the physical, psychological and social problems confronting the elderly and offering advice on how to prevent and deal with them, the Foundation offers a simple but comprehensive resource to seniors. The book was written in question-and-answer format with a detailed index to help readers go directly to the questions they have in mind. This book offers general directions and ideas and should not be considered a substitute for medical attention.

The Foundation is indebted to the generous support we have received from the various foundations in our community that allowed this book to be distributed free of charge in the Quad-City area. We are specifically thankful to the Bechtel Trusts and Foundation, Cardiovascular Medicine, P.C., Genesis Medical Center, Rock Island Community Foundation, and the Scott County Regional Authority. We are also indebted to the tireless effort of many individuals who have made this book a reality by providing a high level of expertise, passion and dedication. I would like to acknowledge Suzanne Hartung and Jan Harper for their tireless editing of the book, Lynne Majetic for the cover design, illustrations and graphic design/layout, and all the MCRF Foundation staff for their efforts and contributions. We also extend special thanks for our Foundation legal and accounting advisers, Mr. Richard Bittner and Mr. Steven Landauer, for their tireless efforts and support to the Foundation.

We sincerely hope that this book will help seniors "keep the fight" and enjoy independence and excellent health.

Nicolas W. Shammas, MD, MS, FACC, FACP
President and Research Director
Midwest Cardiovascular Research Foundation

The Epidemiology of an Aging Population
Jon H. Lemke, PhD, and Amanda K. DeGraeve, BS

What is epidemiology?

Epidemiology is the branch of medicine that deals with the causes, distribution and control of disease in populations. In this chapter, we will focus on the epidemiology of the aging U.S. population.

What is the current U.S. population?

The *U.S. population* reached 300 million in October of 2006 (6.6% growth in 6.5 years). According to the 2000 *U.S. Census*, there were over 281 million people (138 million males and 143 million females) living in the United States. Population estimates are also available on the U.S. Census website.

The following Summary File 1 from the 2000 U.S. Census appears as an eroded pyramid (See Figure 1). There were more people in the 35-39 age group than any other age group. From age group 35-39 plus, there are more females than males in each age group. However, less than age 35 there were 2,778,118 more males than females. There were approximately 14 million males aged 65 years and older and 21 million females aged 65 years and older. Of the individuals aged 55-64, there were 92 males to every 100 females; of those 65-74, there were 82 males to every 100 females; of those 75-84 years, there were 65 males to every 100 females; and of those aged 85 and above, there were 41 males to every 100 females. It is the erosion of the pyramid that has a tremendous impact on public policy and the projections of the costs and viability of government programs.

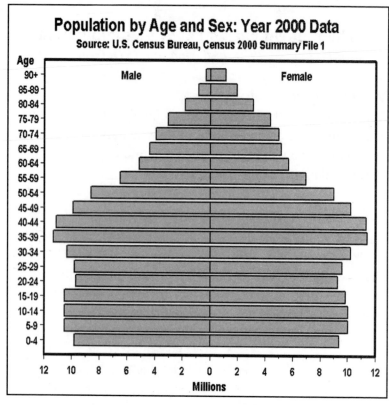

Figure 1. Summary file 1 from the U.S. Census, "Eroded Pyramid."

Of the individuals aged 65 years of age and older, 56% were married and 31% were widowed. The U.S. Census recognizes that **race** and **ethnicity** are different and that people can be combinations of races. Ethnicity is reported as Hispanic/Latino (35.3 million, 12.5% of the population) or not. Of those with at least one race as white, 8.6% were Hispanic/Latino, which is 3 times greater than that of Black/African Americans (2.8%) and Asians (2.7%) *(see Table 1)*. Many other U.S. Census perspectives are available by visiting http://www.census.gov/main/www/cen2000.html.

Table 1: Ethnicity by Race of the U.S. Population from the 2000 U.S. Census

Race Alone or in Combination*	Population Size (2000)	Percent Hispanic/ Latino
White alone or in combination	216,930,975	8.6%
Black or African American alone or in combination	36,419,434	2.8%
American Indian and Alaska Native alone or in combination	4,119,301	16.4%
Asian alone or in combination	11,898,828	2.7%
Native Hawaiian and Other Pacific Islander alone or in combination	874,414	14.4%
Some other race alone or in combination	18,521,486	90.4%
Total population (all races)	281,421,906	12.5%

*Since races are reported in combination, the sum of the race populations is greater than the total population.

The U.S. population reached 300 million in October of 2006 (6.6% growth in 6.5 years). The *rate of growth* is a combination of *mortality rate*, *birth rate*, and *immigration rate*. Many states have now experienced consecutive years with more children graduating from high school than entering kindergarten.

What is the predicted U.S. population for the future?

Predictions of the U.S. population depend upon assumptions about the *mortality rate*, the *birth rate*, and *immigration rate*. The mortality rate is dependent upon estimates of life expectancy.

When a child was born in 1950, the life expectancy of the child was 68.2 years of age. When a child was born in 2004, the life expectancy had increased to 77.9 years of age. The *Social Security Administration* has predicted when a child is born in 2075, the life expectancy will be 81.2 for males and 85 for females. This prediction from the Social Security Administration is conservative compared to others with higher estimates of future life expectancies.

The *National Institute on Aging* estimates that the total U.S. population will grow by approximately 20% by 2030. The *Administration on Aging* estimates that the total U.S. population will grow by approximately 49% by 2050, while the population 65 years of age and older will grow by 147% from the year 2000.

SOURCES: National Institute on Aging - retrieved on 5/5/2006 for 2030 from http://www.nia.nih.gov/NewsAndEvents/PressReleases/PR2006030965PlusReport.htm)
Administration of Aging - retrieved on 5/5/2006 for 2050 from http://www.aoa.gov/press/did_you_know/did_you_know.asp)

What is the difference between life expectancy and life span?

Initially, *life expectancy* is the average length of life for infants born at a given point in time, but as the group survivors age, then the life expectancy continues to increase.

However, *life span* is the maximum age that someone could reach. Currently, the modern day documented life span is 122 years and 164 days as set by *Jeanne Calment* when she died in August of 1997. Others claim to have lived longer, but documentation is lacking. The life expectancy has been increasing without an increase in life span. When some disagree with predicted future increases in life expectancy, they often are expecting the life span to increase rapidly.

What is the impact of lifestyle on one's life expectancy?

The elderly population has been getting more active over the years. Jeanne Calment was very active and still riding her bicycle at 100 years old. Twenty-one percent of older Americans engage in regular physical activities, including walking, weight lifting, fishing, golfing, gardening and swimming.

People make major choices that influence how "fast they age." By the time high school classmates reach the age of 55, some look old enough to be the parents of others . . . and, for all practical purposes, they physically really are! Smokers age faster, married people age slower and diet plays a complex major role. A diet that can be very good for one person could be very bad for another. Conventional wisdom about diet is continually changing and you have to find a diet that works best for you.

Lifestyle goes beyond smoking, diet, physical activity and marriage. Other lifestyle choices that affect the rate of aging include how people supplement their diet with vitamins, challenge their mind, deal with stress, sleep, care for dental needs, maintain good hygiene, interact with a social support network, eliminate risks of accidents, minimize medications, have an active monogamous sex life and maintain a spiritual perspective on life.

Dr. Michael F. Roizen refers to their ***RealAge*** vs. their chronological age and has established the website www.realage.com so people can estimate their own RealAge. His work supports the dominance of lifestyle over genetics in determining one's life expectancy.

Even though one may be genetically susceptible for various medical conditions, one still has influence on the age of onset and the rate of change in severity of illness.

SOURCES: Dramatic changes in US aging highlighted in new census, NIH report. (2006, March 9). Retrieved on November 29, 2006 from http://www. census.gov/Press-Release/www/releases/archives/aging_population/006544.html. Administration on Aging. Retrieved on May 5, 2006 from http://www.aoa.gov/ press/did_you_know/did_you_know.asp.
Roizen, M.F. (2000), RealAge are you as young as you feel? New York, NY: HarperCollins Publishers, Inc.

Can changes in lifestyle improve one's health?

While some of the effects of lifestyle can be seen at 55 and 65 years of age, it is not too late to halt or in some cases reverse the impact of many choices as long as the potential medical problems have not yet occurred.

Many of the adults not participating in physical activities are limited due to chronic and ***comorbid*** conditions (that is, two or more chronic health conditions). The most common conditions that make it difficult and painful for adults to participate in physical activities are arthritis, hypertension, heart disease, diabetes and respiratory disorders.

The inability for many elderly to be physically active contributes to the overweight and obese population. In the U.S., 73% of males and 66% of females 65 and older are overweight. Of those people, 27% of males and 32% of females are obese. The following studies highlight how much lifestyle changes can affect how one ages.

- Irregular heartbeat (cardiac dysrhythmia)
- Anemias
- Solid tumor without metastasis
- Congestive heart failure
- . Hypothyroidism
- Hardening of the arteries (peripheral vascular disease)

SOURCE: Top 10 Comorbidities. Retrieved on May 8, 2006 from http:\\www. ahrq.gov/data/hcup/factbk1/fctbk2.htm.

What are the major causes of death in the U.S.?

The top 15 causes of death in the United States are as follows:

1. Heart disease
2. Cancer
3. Stroke
4. Chronic lower respiratory diseases
5. Accidents
6. Diabetes
7. Alzheimer's disease
8. Influenza and pneumonia
9. Kidney disease
10. Septicemia (overwhelming infection)
11. Suicide
12. Chronic liver disease and cirrhosis
13. High blood pressure and hypertension-related kidney disease
14. Parkinson's disease
15. Pneumonitis (lung inflammation) due to solids and liquids

For individuals 65 years of age and older, the major causes of death include:

1. Heart disease
2. Cancer
3. Stroke
4. Chronic lower respiratory diseases

5. Influenza and pneumonia
6. Diabetes mellitus

SOURCE: Hitti M. (2006, April 19). New record for US life expectancy. Retrieved May 4, 2006 from http:\\www.webmd.com/content/article/121/114175. htm. Center for Disease Control, National Center for Health Statistics

What are the last weeks and days of life commonly like?

Perhaps surprisingly for some, many people appear in good health the week before they die. Many never enter a nursing home, and of those that do, many are there only temporarily to recover from an acute condition. The average age of those who enter a nursing home is 83 years of age.

The events that occur during the last days of life vary from person to person. There are a variety of signs that typically give a good indication that death is approaching. When ***signs of death*** begin to appear, this is called the ***pre-active phase of dying*** and may last up until two weeks prior to the actual time of death. Some of the signs that do indicate the pre-active phase are:

- Pause in breathing
- Restlessness
- Increased need for sleep
- Difficulty healing
- Seeing deceased people

Additional signs that occur approximately three days prior to death include:

- Mottling or blotchy coloring of the skin
- Blue coloration
- Blurred vision
- Incontinence
- Congested or irregular breathing
- Confusion

SOURCE: Making your loved one comfortable during the last days of life. Retrieved on November 29, 2006 from http://www.mayoclinci.com/health/cancer/ CA00048

Where do the last days of life commonly take place?

Preferences vary as to where people want to spend their *last days of life*. When the time comes, you may or may not have a choice. But, you do want your preferences known. You may stay in one of the following:

- Your own home or that of a family member, and receive home health care by family members and healthcare professionals
- A nursing home
- A hospital
- A hospice care center. *Hospice* is care received that will make you as comfortable and pain-free as possible, as well as providing emotional and spiritual support from your care delivery team.

It is important to discuss and share your input as to where you would like your last days of life to be located. Many people wait until it is too late and their family has to guess where their loved one would like to be. Discuss it well in advance of death to assure that your wishes are taken into account.

SOURCE: Center for Disease Control, National Center for Health Statistics.

Chapter 2

Heart Disease as We Grow Older
Nicolas W. Shammas, MD, MS, FACC, FACP

What is heart disease and how it is affected by aging?

Heart disease is a non-specific term that describes all kinds of problems that affect the blood vessels, muscles and electrical system of the heart. Heart disease is more prevalent as we grow older. For instance, *coronary atherosclerosis*, or build-up of plaques in the blood vessels of the heart, is present in over 70% of people over the age of 40 and almost 90% of people over the age of 50 as documented by *ultrasound imaging* inside the blood vessels of the heart. This might not show on an *angiogram* test, an invasive procedure that requires the injection of a contrast dye directly into the blood vessels of the heart. Although these blockages can be very minor and do not result in symptoms, they are likely to rupture, leading to an abrupt closure of the blood vessel of the heart and subsequently a heart attack.

With age, there is also a higher frequency of *hypertension* (65% of people over the age of 60), and *diabetes* (18.3% of people over the age of 60); conditions associated with *plaque build-up* in the coronaries, weaker heart muscle (or *cardiomyopathy*) and *heart failure*.

In addition, *degenerative changes to the electrical system* of the heart occur more frequently with age, quite often leading to the need for a *pacemaker* implantation. Finally, *degenerative changes in the heart valves* can occur, leading to a severe leak or narrowing in these valves, requiring valve change or repair.

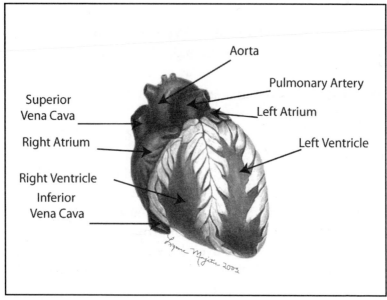

Figure 1.
Heart with major external structures

How frequent is heart disease?

Heart disease affects 22 million people in the United States, or about 10.9% of the total population. It remains the number one killer in our country, costing our healthcare system over $300 billion dollars annually. On average, 930 Americans die daily from a ***heart attack***, or a sudden interruption of blood supply to part of the heart muscle. Over 60 million people in the United States are at high risk of ***heart failure***. Five million people live with heart failure, a condition caused by weakness or excessive stiffness of the heart muscle, leading to shortness of breath, reduced energy level, fatigue, swelling of the lower extremities and occasionally chest pain.

What are the risk factors of coronary artery disease?

Coronary artery disease (CAD) is plaque build-up in the blood vessels of the heart. Risk factors for CAD are classified as major or minor. Major ones include *hypertension*, *diabetes*, *cigarette smoking*, *abnormal lipids* (such as *cholesterol* and *triglycerides*), *obesity*, and *genetic factors*. Minor risk factors include *age*, *lack of physical activity* and *gender*. The majority of these risk factors with the exception of age, gender and genetics are modifiable by *lifestyle changes*, *diet*, *exercise*, *weight control* or *medicine*. Age as noted is a minor risk factor and therefore growing older is not necessarily equivalent to having heart disease but does require that a more aggressive approach to controlling modifiable risk factors should be taken.

How does a heart attack occur?

A *heart attack* indicates a sudden interruption of the blood supply to a part of the heart muscle due to an abrupt blockage in the blood vessel (*coronary artery*) that supplies it. Blockages can be very minor and still lead to heart attacks. In fact, more than 60% of heart attacks occur in blockages which are less than 50% in severity that cannot be detected by stress testing. These blockages are also typically not subjected to treatment with *balloon angioplasty* as they do not produce a lack of blood supply to the heart in normal conditions and do not cause symptoms.

Angioplasty, or stretching of the blockage with a balloon or a stainless steel mesh called *stent*, has not been shown to reduce the chance of a heart attack in patients with stable symptoms. Its only purpose is to reduce symptoms of chest pain and shortness of breath and reduce the use of cardiac drugs.

A *heart attack* leads to scarring of a part of the heart muscle. This happens within a few hours of the artery blocked. However, within the first hour of symptoms, the heart is at risk of *electrical instability* that can lead to a *cardiac arrest,* or the inability of the heart to pump blood to the body and the brain. Cardiac arrest results in death if not corrected within minutes by shocking the heart with a *defibrillator* to its original heart rhythm.

Patients who experience *sudden chest pain* or *shortness of breath* need to seek immediate medical attention by calling **9-1-1** and **NOT** driving themselves to the hospital. A heart attack is best treated by proceeding immediately to the *cardiac catheterization laboratory*, where the artery is treated immediately with an *angioplasty*. Current guidelines encourage opening a closed artery in the setting of the heart attack within 90 minutes of arrival to the emergency room. *The sooner the heart attack is aborted, the more muscle is saved in the heart and the longer a person lives.*

What is angina?

Angina is chest pain that results from a narrowing in one of the blood vessels of the heart leading to reduction of oxygen to this part of the heart muscle. *Stable angina* is chest pain that occurs during exertion when the heart is in high demand for oxygen. Typically, stable angina is predictable at a certain level of activity, does not occur at rest and resolves within few minutes of rest or *sublingual nitroglycerin*. It is generally located in the middle of the chest (mid sternal) but can also occur from the mid abdomen all the way to the jaw and can radiate to the arms, neck and back. Stable angina might not be apparent in many patients and is silent particularly in diabetics. Females frequently have an atypical pattern of chest pain that can be difficult to link to the heart. A low threshold to evaluate chest pain in a female is needed, particularly in seniors with several cardiac risk factors.

In contrast to stable angina, *unstable angina* is lack of blood supply to the heart at rest and is generally due to an unstable plaque within the blood vessel of the heart, probably ruptured but which did not lead to a complete interruption of the blood supply. This type of blockage can lead to a full heart attack if not attended to immediately. Generally a clot forms over the blockage and can expand to block the artery completely. A patient needs to be admitted to the hospital, and treatment with blood thinners including aspirin, Plavix (clopidogrel), and heparin or heparin-like products is generally immediately initiated. Also, nitroglycerin intravenously is initiated to prevent spasm over the narrowed artery and dilate the blood vessels of the heart. Also, nitroglycerin reduces the work load on the heart and reduces oxygen needed by the heart. Other medications are also used, including **beta blockers** or **calcium channel blockers,** that will be discussed in detail in another chapter of this book. The ultimate treatment of unstable angina is an angiogram and angioplasty of the blocked artery. It is highly recommended that this be done within 48 hours of admission to the hospital.

How do blockages in the heart get diagnosed?

Most often the suspicion for severe blockages in the heart vessels occurs while taking a history from the patient. Patients that describe chest pressure or pain with exertion that resolves with rest and have multiple cardiac risk factors have a high likelihood of blockages in their coronaries particularly if they are over the age of 55. These patients quite often undergo **angiography** (as described below) to further define the presence of blockages in their coronary arteries.

The diagnosis of coronary disease is generally more challenging, however, as more than half the patients do not have typical symptoms. A **stress test** is then performed before proceeding with an angiogram to help identify patients who are likely to have significant blockages in their coronaries. A stress test can be performed in many ways, including walking on a ***treadmill*** or by injecting a medicine in a patient's arm vein that chemically stresses the heart, such as ***adenosine*** or ***dobutamine***.

Changes in the electricity of the heart are monitored during the stress test by obtaining ***serial electrocardiograms*** that could indirectly point toward blockages in the coronaries. In addition to monitoring the electrical conduction of the heart, monitoring of the blood supply by nuclear imaging or the motion of the heart muscle by ***echocardiography*** (ultrasound pictures of the heart) under stress enhances the accuracy of identifying blockages in the coronaries.

What is an angiogram?

An ***angiogram*** or a ***cardiac catheterization*** is an ***invasive test*** that requires placing a plastic tube from the groin to the heart blood vessels. A ***contrast dye*** is injected inside the blood vessels, showing their insides and revealing whether blockages are present. The angiogram shows the inside of the blood vessel (***lumen***) but not what is in the wall of the vessel. It is like looking at the "donut hole, not the donut itself." Blockages can be present, but if they are not protruding inside the lumen of the vessel, they might not be seen on an angiogram. These blockages can cause heart attacks, as noted above, as they can rupture and cause a sudden ***blood clot*** that closes the artery.

What is an angioplasty?

An ***angioplasty*** indicates treatment of a blockage inside a blood vessel by stretching the ***artery*** (to the most part) and compressing the ***blockage*** (to a much lesser degree) using a ***balloon*** or a ***stent***. The balloon is inflated under high pressure to compress the area of the blockage. A stent is a stainless steel or cobalt mesh that is inflated by a balloon stretching a vessel wall and not allowing it to recoil back or tear. Stents currently in use are loaded with medications that work to prevent scar tissue from occurring at the site of the treatment as part of the healing process. These are called ***Drug Eluting Stents (DES)***. When a DES stent is deployed, a patient should take a ***combination blood thinner*** (***aspirin*** and ***clopidogrel***) for a period of at least a year after stenting to prevent clotting from forming on the metal part of the stent.

Other methods of treating blockages in the artery of the heart include ***rotational atherectromy,*** or the use of a burr coated with diamond dust to remove blockages at high rotational speed, or ***directional atherectomy***, the use of a cutter to cut the plaque and remove it from the artery. All these methods are very effective in reducing the plaque burden inside the artery but continue to provide inferior historic results compared to the DES.

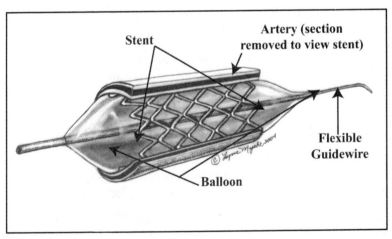

Figure 2.
Stent mounted on a balloon being implanted in an artery

What is bypass surgery?

Bypass surgery is a procedure that requires taking a vein from the leg or an artery from under the collar bone and attaching them from the *aorta*, the main artery that comes out of the heart, to the main blood vessels of the heart past areas of blockages, therefore literally *bypassing* the blocked blood vessel and restoring normal blood supply to the heart muscle. Bypass surgery is performed in patients with severe and complex blockages that cannot be treated with angioplasty. Serious risks of the surgery vary with centers and operators' experience and patients' comorbid risk factors such as, stroke, bleeding, infection, heart attack, death and others. There have been fewer bypasses performed in the United States since the advent of medicated stents, as interventional cardiologists can now tackle longer and more complex blockages with better outcomes with angioplasty.

What is cardiac rehabilitation?

Cardiac rehabilitation is an exercise program administered to cardiac patients with history of blockages in their heart arteries and who have undergone angioplasty or surgery. Also, patients with *valve surgeries* and *congestive heart failure* can benefit significantly from a *structured exercise program*.

Cardiac rehabilitation starts in the hospital. Phase I starts before the patient is discharged. The goal is to get the patient to start exercise immediately after surgery and be independent before leaving for home. Added to this is an educational program about prevention of heart disease, including nutritional information.

Phase II starts shortly after the patient leaves the hospital and is conducted under a close monitoring of patient's heart rhythm and blood pressure and under the supervision of experienced rehabilitation staff. It lasts about 8-12 weeks and prepares the patient for a more intense and independent exercise program that can be performed with minimal or no supervision (Phase III and Phase IV).

Cardiac rehabilitation has been shown to improve patients' self-confidence, quality and probably quantity of life. It also reduces the chance of depression and allows a patient to resume full functional life shortly after surgery.

What is pericarditis?

Pericarditis, or inflammation around the lining of the heart, can be triggered by infections, inflammatory diseases, radiation to the chest, tumors, heart attacks, trauma, kidney failure, thyroid disease and cardiac surgeries. It can happen at any age. The *pericardium* is a strong sac that surrounds the heart. It has many functions, including producing a lubricant, protecting against infections and preventing sudden stretching and enlargement of the heart. Pericarditis can be treated by pain killers and anti-inflammatory drugs. It typically presents itself with a sharp, mid sternal chest pain that seems to get worse when a person lays flat and get better when a person sits forward. A characteristic rub is generated from the inflamed pericardium and can be detected by a *stethoscope* in a doctor's office. An inflamed pericardium can lead to more scarring and thickness in the lining of the heart, constricting the ability of the heart to expand and causing shortness of breath and heart failure. This could be treated with surgical stripping of the pericardium.

What is cardiomyopathy?

Cardiomyopathy is a disorder of the heart muscle itself. It often is due to an *intrinsic heart muscle problem* (*primary cardiomyopathy*) or it can be acquired (*secondary cardiomyopathy*) by *viral infections*, lack of blood supply to the heart, long-standing high blood pressure and diabetes, excess alcohol intake, pregnancy, chemotherapeutic drugs, and infiltrative diseases of the heart that can penetrate and deposit in the heart muscle. Cardiomyopathy leads to *excess weakness of the heart muscle* (*systolic dysfunction*) or *stiffness of the heart muscle* (*diastolic dysfunction*). It can cause heart failure with build-up of fluid in the lungs, shortness of breath, inability to lie down flat and sudden shortness of breath that awakens the patient from sleep.

Primary cardiomyopathy is classified into *dilated*, *restrictive* and *hypertrophic*. *Dilated cardiomyopathy (DCM)* is more prevalent in patients over the age of 55. It is characterized by enlargement of all the cavities of the heart. It mostly leads to weakness of the heart muscle and heart failure. Treatment of DCM consists of a combination of medications including *beta blockers*, *angiotension converting ace inhibitors*, *digoxin* and *aldosterone blockers*. If the heart function reaches a low level (ejection fraction less than 35%), an *internal defibrillator* is implanted to protect the heart against lethal arrhythmias. Also, *biventricular pacemakers* are implanted in these patients that fail medical treatment to help improve their symptoms and reduce the recurrences of congestive heart failure.

What is heart failure?

Heart failure (HF) is defined as the inability of the heart to pump adequate amount of blood to meet the oxygen demands of the body. This can be the result of either weakness or excessive stiffness of the heart muscle. In either situation, the pressure inside the heart increases leading to shortness of breath, fluid in the lungs, fluid retention and occasionally swelling in the lower extremities.

HF has multiple risk factors, including blockages in the

arteries of the heart, viral infection to the muscle of the heart, high blood pressure (or hypertension), diabetes, anemia, excess alcohol intake, severe leak or narrowing in some of the valves of the heart, various systemic diseases such as inflammatory disorders and deposits of various proteins in the muscle of the heart (infiltrative diseases) and family history of weak heart muscle (cardiomyopathy). As we grow older, many of these risk factors become more prevalent and the incidence of heart failure increases.

Stiff heart muscle also increases with age and is more common in older women than older men.

The treatment of the heart failure consists of targeting the cause of the failure, removing any excess fluid with diuretics and in the case of a weak heart muscle, placing the patient on a combination of drugs that includes beta blockers, ace inhibitors and aldosterone inhibitors.

Stiff heart muscle is treated with aggressive management of blood pressure, as well as the use of drugs that relax the heart and reduce heart thickness over time.

HF patients are monitored with frequent blood checks to monitor their blood potassium and sodium and kidney function and by checking heart strength with non-invasive imaging to monitor response to drug therapy and stability of the heart strength over time. Current therapy has improved the prognosis of patients with HF. However, HF incidence continues to be on the rise because of the increase in obesity incidence in the U.S. and subsequent high blood pressure and diabetes, both major risk factors for HF. Therefore, HF management starts with improving lifestyle and dietary interventions and exercise and reducing obesity incidence.

How does aging affect the heart valves?

The heart has four *valves*. The two valves that separate between the lower (*ventricles*) and top (*atria*) chambers of the heart are called the *mitral* and *tricuspid valves*, and the heart valves that separate between the ventricles and the great vessels that arise out of the heart are called the *aortic* and *pulmonic valves*. The two valves that are commonly affected by aging are the mitral and aortic valve. As we grow older, excess scar tissue and calcium deposit on these heart valves. This might lead to narrowing and/or severe leak in the valves, reducing the amount of blood leaving the heart to various body organs and exerting a lot of stress on the heart itself. Narrowing in the mitral valve can cause significant shortness of breath and under exertion can cause chest pain or loss of consciousness. A leaky aortic valve can cause

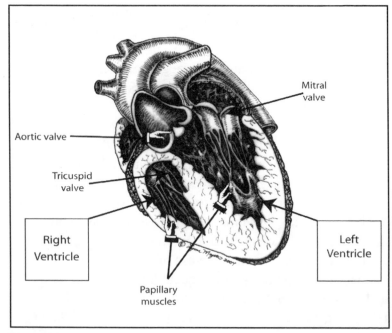

Figure 3.
Heart Valves (Pulmonic valve not seen due to plane of dissection)

primarily shortness of breath and congestive heart failure. A narrowed aortic valve can cause shortness of breath, chest pain, fainting spells and congestive heart failure. As both mitral and aortic valves leak, stress on the heart becomes significant and the heart stretches and weakens. Pressure inside the heart also increases and the patient becomes short of breath and heart failure develops. Treatment of the valves can be with medications, but as symptoms appear despite medical treatment, or early signs of heart stretching and weakness become evident, valve repair or replacement becomes necessary. Your physician decides on the type of valve you might need whether it is a tissue valve or a mechanical valve. This takes into consideration whether you have a contraindication to a ***blood thinner*** (namely ***warfarin***), as this is required for mechanical valves, or based on your age, life expectancy or the presence of preexistent rhythm disturbances. Currently, the majority of mitral valves can be repaired, reducing the need for valve replacement and keeping a patient's native valve.

How can we protect our heart valves against infection?

Damaged heart valves or abnormal heart valves can be prone to infection, a condition called bacterial ***endocarditis***. This condition damages the valves fast and leads to various complications including severe ***leak in the valves*** or ***vegetations on the valves***. Vegetations are growth of bacteria or fungus on the valves that can eventually chip off and migrate to the head or other organs in the body, leading to various complications including abscesses, strokes and widespread infection. If you know you have an abnormal heart valve, you need to let your dentist, urologist or gastroenterologist be aware of this. Procedures to the oral cavity such as teeth cleaning, or to the bladder or the stomach/colon such as an endoscope procedure or a biopsy, can lead to transient bacteria into the blood stream which can lead to infection of the damaged or abnormal heart valve. This can be easily prevented by an antibiotic that can be taken approximately one hour prior to the procedure that your physician performing the procedure orders for you.

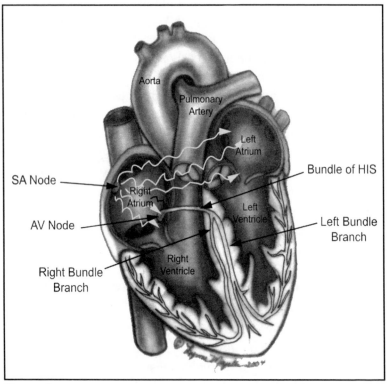

Figure 4.
Electrical system of the heart

What are the common causes of fainting in the elderly?

The causes of *fainting* (*syncope*) are varied but can be easily classified into *cardiovascular* (generated from the heart and blood vessels), *neurologic* (generated from the central nervous system, such as the brain) and *neurogenic* (an imbalance in the control of the tone of the blood vessels).

On occasion, the causes of fainting remain unknown despite all tests performed to clarify its origin. This can be very frustrating to both the physician and the patient and unfortunately occurs in about 20% of patients. About 7% of these patients will have recurrences of fainting with continued unknown reasons.

Cardiac reasons for fainting include ***abnormal heart rhythms***, such as a very fast or slow heart beat due to either lack of blood supply to the heart; ***congenital abnormalities*** (in the heart muscle, the valves or the electrical wiring of the heart); ***degenerative changes*** to the electrical wiring of the heart; or abnormal electrolytes such as calcium or potassium in the blood stream. ***Severe narrowing in the valves*** of the heart can also lead to fainting spells. Typically a cardiac evaluation includes an ***ultrasound*** to the heart to evaluate the valves and muscle of the heart, a ***stress test*** to exclude blockages in the blood vessels of the heart, and a ***monitor*** that can continuously monitor and record the heart beats for 24 to 48 hours (***Holter monitor***) or intermittently record the heart rhythm on demand by the patient (***Event care monitor***). Blood tests to check for the electrolytes and thyroid functions are also obtained.

Neurologic causes of syncope include ***seizure disorder***, ***strokes*** and ***severe migraines***. The neurologist typically evaluates this condition with a thorough neurological exam, an MRI or CT scan of the heart and an ***electroencephalogram (EEG)*** to rule out abnormal brain wave activity such as a seizure disorder.

Neurogenic fainting or **near-fainting spells** are caused by an imbalance in the nervous system that controls the tone of the blood vessels of the body. Patients typically experience these dizzy spells after they have been standing or sitting for longer times, are dehydrated, have been in excessively warm surroundings or after heavy exertion. Typically, dizziness or fainting spells are preceded by a feeling of nausea and the patient can generally predict that he or she will become dizzy or faint. This condition can be diagnosed with a ***Tilt Table test***. During this test, a patient lies down on a table that is tilted 80 degrees after being strapped appropriately. The heart rhythm and blood pressure are carefully monitored. Medications are administered to simulate conditions that could provoke neurogenic dizziness. The test is positive if it reproduces the patient's symptoms and alters the blood pressure and heart rate accordingly. If diagnosed, this condition is treatable mostly by preventative measures such as avoiding excess heat, standing or sitting for long hours and heavy exertion. If the feeling of dizziness occurs, lying down and having the feet slightly above the head reverses this condition within a few minutes. Medications such as beta blockers are also very effective in reducing the intensity of this condition.

Other causes of dizziness or fainting spells also include a ***hypersensitive spot in the carotid bulb***, located in the neck blood vessel (***carotid artery***). Rubbing or stretching the neck in some patients can stimulate this spot that controls the tone of the blood vessels in the body leading to slowing of the heart rate and a drop in blood pressure. This leads to fainting or severe dizziness. In addition, ***orthostatic drop in blood pressure*** occurs when a person abruptly stands up from a lying down or sitting position and can lead to significant dizzy spells or even transient fainting. This is common in diabetics, dehydrated patients and patients on various cardiac medications. It is also made worse by certain medical conditions including weak heart muscle (***cardiomyopathy***).

What are arrhythmias?

An ***arrhythmia*** is defined as an ***electrical disturbance of the*** *heart*. A very common arrhythmia is *skipped beats*. This is generally benign but sometimes can be precipitated by serious conditions such as *thickening of the heart muscle (hypertrophy), electrolyte disturbance, valvular problem, thyroid disease*, or *lack of blood supply to the heart*.

Another common arrhythmia is *atrial fibrillation*, highly prevalent in the elderly population. This electrical disturbance is due to a chaotic heart rhythm that is generated from the top portion of the heart (*atria*). It is characterized by a *fast, irregular heart beat*. The danger of this heart rhythm is *stroke* or a *weak heart muscle* (*cardiomyopathy*). Patients with this condition are typically treated with *warfarin*, a blood thinner, and medications that control the heart speed (*beta blockers* or *digoxin*). Other aggressive therapies include an invasive procedure that isolates the source of the irregular heart beat by either a *high energy radiofrequency current* or *cryoablation (freezing)* of the source of the arrhythmia. *Pacemaker therapy* can be a part of the treatment of this condition.

In addition, many conditions, including prior heart attacks, blockages in the artery of the heart, certain drugs, electrolyte abnormalities, severe narrowing or leak in the heart valves, a weak heart muscle or cardiomyopathy can result in an abnormal heart rhythm generated from the bottom portion of the heart called *ventricular tachycardia*. This generally leads to a very fast heart beat, a drop in blood pressure and fainting spells. Ventricular tachycardia can also degenerate into *ventricular fibrillation*, where the heart's electrical system becomes chaotic and ceases to pump blood to the vital organs of the body. This leads to cardiac arrest and death if not corrected immediately and within 4-5 minutes, typically by delivering an electrical shock to the heart (*defibrillation*) to abort the abnormal electrical conduction. This condition can be treated with medications or an implantable internal defibrillator.

Finally, elderly people are at risk of a ***degenerative change in the electrical system of the heart*** leading to slowing of the heart beat that necessitates a ***pacemaker implantation***. A pacemaker generates an electrical impulse to the heart in a rhythmic way stimulating the heart muscle to conduct electricity at a rate similar to the normal heart conduction.

You can be alerted to an electrical disturbance of the heart by watching for the following symptoms: ***a flutter in the chest, irregular heart beat, near-fainting or fainting spells, sudden shortness of breath, chest pain, confusion, unexplained fatigue and tiredness***. If you experience any of these symptoms, you need to undergo an evaluation by your physician. Although some of these symptoms can be caused by other medical conditions, a cardiac source needs to be ruled out.

Heart disease accounts for about half of all deaths as we grow older. Many of these problems are preventable irrespective of age. Clearly, ***exercise, quitting smoking, maintaining an ideal body weight, balanced nutrition with low fat and a high content of fibers, vegetables and fruits,*** as well as a ***better management of inevitable daily stresses,*** are very important measures to help fight heart disease. In addition, ***routine medical check-ups*** to monitor for high blood pressure, diabetes and high blood fat and treat them aggressively are critical steps in fighting against heart disease progression.

Chapter 3

Peripheral Vascular Disease
Eric J. Dippel, MD

What is Peripheral Vascular Disease?
Peripheral vascular disease (PVD) is a term that describes blockages in the blood vessels that supply the entire body except the neck and head (called *cerebrovascular disease*) and the heart (called *coronary artery disease*).

Cholesterol not only clogs the arteries of the heart, but also clogs other arteries in the body. All of the arteries in the body are susceptible to this problem. The arteries to the neck, called the *carotid arteries*, supply the head. When the carotid arteries become significantly blocked, patients are susceptible to a *stroke.*

The arteries to the kidneys, known as the *renal arteries*, also frequently become blocked. Typically, there are no symptoms associated with *renal artery narrowing*. The kidneys are one of the organs that control *blood pressure*; therefore, a sudden increase in blood pressure might be a sign that the kidney arteries are becoming blocked.

When blockage occurs in the legs in a mild or moderate degree, the most common symptom is *claudication*, a tight or tired sensation in the leg muscles that occurs with walking and is relieved with rest. When the blockages to the leg's arteries become severe enough, then tissue in the leg begins to develop ulcers and die. If blood flow is not re-established promptly, then patients may require *amputation* of part of their leg.

What are the risk factors for Peripheral Vascular Disease (PVD)?

The risk factors for *peripheral vascular disease (PVD)* are identical to the *risk factors of coronary artery disease (CAD)*. This includes high cholesterol, cigarette smoking, diabetes, high blood pressure, obesity and a family history of vascular disease. Since the risk factors for PVD and CAD are the same, many patients have both problems at the same time. Patients with PVD most likely die from heart attacks and strokes rather than from blockages in their lower legs. PVD typically gets worse as people get older. The arteries in the body become blocked over time. Among the above risk factors, smoking is the most hazardous for patients with PVD. Quitting smoking not only reduces the risk of further disease, but also can be one of the most important interventions that can be done to reduce symptoms of pain in the lower legs.

How common is PVD?

PVD is actually extremely common. It is frequently under-recognized and under-diagnosed. A very simple analogy is: When Grandpa walks to the mailbox and gets chest pain, he is referred to the emergency room. However, when Grandpa walks to the mailbox and his legs get tired, he simply is told he is "getting too old." Millions of Americans have PVD, yet only a few are actually being treated. Furthermore, there are thousands of amputations performed in this country every year that might be prevented if the blockages obstructing the blood flow to the leg were treated earlier. There are over 12 million people in the USA that live with peripheral vascular disease. Less than 25% are being treated. A higher index of suspicion is necessary for both patients and physicians to adequately search for, diagnose and treat PVD.

What is Claudication?

Claudication is the symptom of leg fatigue and cramps that patients with PVD describe when they exert themselves. This is typically described as a "tight" or "cramping" sensation in the calves, thighs, or buttocks that occurs with walking. Typically, this occurs at a very predictable time in walking. For example, after walking 1 to 2 blocks, a patient would have to stop and rest. Patients who get cramps in their legs at night while sleeping typically are not experiencing PVD.

What are the causes of leg pain?

Leg pain can be broken down into three major categories:

1. The first category is a problem *with blocked blood vessels* and *poor circulation*. As described above, these symptoms of claudication occur with *walking* or *exertion* and are alleviated with rest. Patients can develop pain that occurs with rest only if the blockages are severe and the blood flow to the leg is extremely limited. Typically, if this occurs, there are other findings, such as *discoloration* of the skin or *ulcerations* of the foot, that go along with resting pain from poor circulation.

2. The second major type of leg pain is due to problems with the bones and joints, such as arthritis of the knees, ankles, and hips. This type of pain is typically worse with standing and weight bearing on the joint. It may occur at rest and not uncommonly, is improved with walking.

3. The third major type of pain is caused by *nerve problems*. For example, pinched nerves in the low back can cause *sciatica pain* which shoots down the hip and buttocks into the lower leg. This pain typically feels sharp and may be worse with certain positions. Another type of nerve pain is numbness

and tingling of the feet that is frequently seen in diabetes. This has a sensation of *"pins and needles"* and may be present 24 hours a day.

What tests can be done to evaluate for PVD?

These tests can be broken down into *noninvasive studies* versus *invasive studies*.

The simplest noninvasive study measures the *blood pressure* in the arms and compares it to the blood pressure in the legs. This is known as the *ankle/brachial index (ABI)*. The blood pressure in the ankles should be roughly the same as the blood pressure in the arms. If the ankle blood pressure is significantly decreased, then this is evidence that there are blockages somewhere in the legs.

Pictures of the arteries in the legs can be obtained through either a *CT scan* or an *MR scan*. While these images are similar, for technical reasons, the CT scan probably provides more accurate images.

Doppler ultrasound also can be used to measure blood flow into the arteries. This test is most commonly used to monitor the *patency of bypass grafts*. An *angiogram* is an invasive test that involves placing a small plastic tube, or *catheter*, into the artery and injecting dye that can be seen with X-ray equipment.

What are the treatments for PVD?

The two most important treatments for PVD are *aggressive risk factor modification* and a *daily walking program*. It is extremely important that the risk factors mentioned above be controlled to prevent these blockages from becoming worse over time. Also, it is extremely important that patients *stop cigarette smoking* and *lower their cholesterol* and *control their diabetes and blood pressure* to normal recommended levels.

Walking is very important to help maintain muscle tone, lower body weight and develop better circulation to the feet. Patients should try to achieve a goal of walking 30 minutes a day, at least 5 days a week. There is one medication that has been approved by the FDA, called Pletal ®, that can help improve blood flow to the feet. Pletal has been shown to increase the distance patients can walk before they develop claudication. For mild claudication, it is a very effective medication. It does not by itself, however, "dissolve" the blockages that are in the arteries, and patients with moderate-to-severe claudication frequently require procedures to open blocked arteries.

What types of procedures can be performed to open blocked arteries in the legs?

Similar to arteries in the heart, arteries in the legs can be opened by using *catheters*, such as balloons and stents, or by surgery to bypass the blocked vessel. Patients typically prefer balloons and stents because this is less invasive. This is called a *percutaneous procedure*, in contrast to the surgical one that requires a bypass. Percutaneous procedures have significantly shorter recovery time with less discomfort, and the long-term outcome results are as good as or better than surgery. Therefore, the first-line approach to opening blocked blood vessels in the legs should be with a balloon or stent if the blockage is amenable to this kind of therapy. If the artery cannot be successfully opened percutaneously, then surgery often is a reasonable alternative.

Why do my legs swell?

Leg swelling, known as *edema*, can be caused by a number of reasons. Some of these problems may be quite serious, while others are rather benign and cosmetic. Swelling in both legs may represent a heart or kidney problem, or a more benign problem is incompetent valves in the veins of the legs (*varicose veins*). Swelling in one leg may represent a ***blood clot*** in that leg or ***a blockage in the lymph nodes*** in the groin. It is also common for a leg to swell after veins have been removed for ***coronary artery bypass grafting***. **Any new swelling of one or both legs should be evaluated by your primary care physician.**

What is abdominal angina?

Abdominal angina is pain in the abdomen resulting from blockages to the main arteries that supply the gut. It typically presents itself with pain in the abdomen after eating that

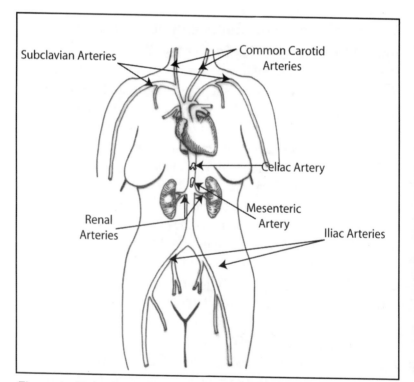

Figure 1. Major Arteries branching from the Aorta.

cannot be explained by gastrointestinal pathology such as gallbladder disease or ulcers or inflammatory diseases. Blockages in those arteries, called the *celiac* or *mesenteric arteries*, can lead to a reduction in the blood supply needed for digestion and transport of food to the body from the gut (See Figure 1). Patients typically experience predictable pain in the abdomen after eating food and subsequently experience weight loss, because they develop an aversion to eating. *Cholesterol plaques* cause a narrowing in these arteries similar to blockages in the neck, heart and legs. Treatment of these blockages can be done with *angioplasty* and *stents*. The diagnosis is best made by a *CT angiogram* or a conventional *angiogram* in the catheterization laboratory. Generally, treatment of these blockages can lead to resolution of symptoms almost immediately after the procedure.

DISEASES OF THE BLOOD VESSELS OF THE HEAD AND NECK

What are the blood vessels that go to the brain?
There are four major blood vessels that go to the brain. The two *carotid arteries* in the front part of the neck can actually be felt pulsating adjacent to your Adam's apple, just below the angle of the jaw. There also are two *vertebral arteries* that go to the back of the brain and run in the bony portion of the spine. These four arteries all connect with each other in the brain.

What is Carotid Artery Disease?
Carotid Artery Disease (CAD) occurs when the *carotid arteries*, like other arteries in the body, become clogged with *cholesterol* over time. The risk factors that cause these blockages include high cholesterol, cigarette smoking,

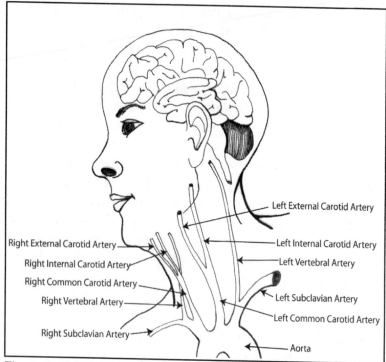

Figure 2. Arteries that supply the head and neck.

diabetes, high blood pressure and family history. When the carotid arteries become severely narrowed, this can lead to decreased blood flow to the brain, which can subsequently lead to a stroke. Carotid artery disease is not associated with pain in the neck or headaches. When the carotid arteries become significantly narrowed, the blood can actually be heard "whooshing" through the blockage when a physician listens to the neck with a stethoscope. This noise is called a *bruit*.

How can atherosclerosis, or blockage in the carotid arteries, be prevented?

The build-up of cholesterol, or *atherosclerosis*, in the carotid arteries occurs for the same reason cholesterol builds up in other arteries of the body. In fact, many patients with *coronary artery disease (CAD)* or *peripheral vascular disease (PVD)* also have carotid disease. Aggressive modification of the risk factors that cause atherosclerosis will prevent the build-up of cholesterol in the arteries. This includes lowering your cholesterol, stopping smoking, controlling diabetes and high blood pressure, maintaining an ideal body weight and getting regular exercise.

What types of tests are used to diagnose Carotid Artery Disease?

The simplest test is merely listening to the neck with a stethoscope for a *bruit*. Sometimes, however, bruits may be difficult to hear. A more accurate noninvasive test is a *carotid Doppler*, which is simply an ultrasound of the blood flow through the neck. *CT scanning* and *MR scanning* can also be helpful in providing three-dimensional images of the carotid and vertebral arteries. Finally, the "gold standard" is an *angiogram*, which is an invasive test where a catheter is inserted in the groin and threaded up to the carotid and vertebral arteries. Contrast dye is injected through the catheter and X-ray movie pictures are taken of the arteries in the neck.

When is it necessary to have a procedure to open the neck arteries?

Whether or not carotid arteries should be treated with a procedure to open them up depends on several factors. One of the primary factors is whether the patient has had a prior symptom, such as a stroke or TIA. The second major factor is the degree of *stenosis* or narrowing in the artery. In combination, these findings have provided a framework to decide if a patient should have a procedure to open the arteries versus simply continuing with medical therapy to prevent further build-up of cholesterol.

How can blocked arteries in the neck be reopened?

Historically, the primary way to open up the carotid arteries is with surgery. This procedure has been performed for approximately 50 years and involves a surgeon cutting open the artery, scraping out the plaque and sewing the artery back together. This procedure is known as a *carotid endarterectomy (CEA)*. Within the past few years, technology has evolved where now the arteries can be opened up with a balloon and a stent via a catheter inserted through the groin under minimally invasive techniques. Recent data comparing carotid stenting versus surgery suggests that in certain high-risk groups of patients, stenting may be superior to surgery. There continue to be ongoing studies looking at lower-risk groups of patients.

What is an aneurysm?

An *aneurysm* is a weakened area of an artery that is bulging out in the same way that a garden hose may develop a bulge at a weak spot. The danger in aneurysms is if they become large enough, they can spontaneously rupture, which will cause bleeding in the brain and a stroke. Aneurysms can occur throughout the body but most commonly occur in the main aorta that runs down through the chest and abdomen. If an aortic aneurysm were to rupture, this could be a life-threatening event. Therefore, aneurysms are typically repaired with surgery or, more recently, with less invasive *stent grafting.* Unfortunately, many times aneurysms do not have any symptoms prior to rupture, other than possible non-specific headaches. Aneurysms are usually a genetic problem, so if there is a family history of aneurysms, it would be worthwhile to be screened for one. Screening for aortic aneurysms can be done using an *abdominal ultrasound* or *CT scan*.

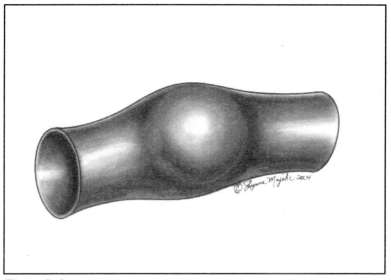

Figure 3. Aneurysm.

What is the treatment for brain aneurysms?

The traditional way to treat *brain aneurysms* was by surgery to clip the aneurysm sac. However, over the last few years, a new treatment has been developed. It is now possible to thread a small catheter up the artery from the groin into the brain and place small coils inside the aneurysm. The advantage of using the catheters is that the recovery time is significantly less and the skull does not have to be opened.

Summing Up . . .

If you smoke, stop! Eat healthfully, maintain an appropriate body weight and get plenty of exercise. If you have high blood pressure, get it under control with a combination of weight loss, healthful eating, exercise and medication, as prescribed by your doctor. If you have a family history of aneurysms, get screened.

Chapter 4

The Aging Brain
Rodney A. Short, MD

Introduction

This chapter is about diseases of aging that affect the brain. The brain is much like the heart and other organs in some respects. Diseases of the blood vessels, infections, cancers, trauma and immune disorders can all affect the brain just as they can affect other parts of the body.

However, the brain is also unique in two respects. First, the symptoms of brain diseases are much more varied than symptoms of diseases of any other organ system. *Numbness, weakness, walking problems, speech difficulty, memory loss, personality change, alteration of consciousness, vision impairment* and *headaches* are just a few of the many symptoms that can reflect a brain disorder.

Second, the brain is susceptible to several intrinsic diseases that do not affect other organ systems.

This chapter will discuss two of these very common diseases, *Alzheimer's* and *Parkinson's*, along with disease of the blood vessels to the brain, also more commonly known as *stroke*.

What is a stroke?

A *stroke* is a sudden disruption in blood supply to the brain. Some health care workers use the term *cerebrovascular accident (or CVA)*, although stroke is now the preferred term.

The blood supply to the brain can be disrupted in two ways. The first is by a lack of blood flow through an artery (or less commonly a vein), which leads to *ischemia to the brain,* or *ischemic stroke*. The other is by a leakage in a blood vessel causing **bleeding into the brain**, or **hemorrhagic stroke**. Disruption of blood flow to the brain can cause symptoms immediately, and irreversible damage to the brain can occur within minutes, which is why time is critical in treating stroke.

What are the symptoms of stroke?

Strokes are like real estate because it's all about location, location, location. Depending on the location of brain affected, any of the symptoms mentioned in the introduction can occur during a stroke. The key to recognizing a stroke is **that symptoms begin suddenly and usually affect one side of body if physical symptoms (such as numbness, weakness) are involved**. Therefore, any sudden numbness, weakness or vision loss on one side of the body or sudden speech problems, dizziness or confusion can signify a stroke.

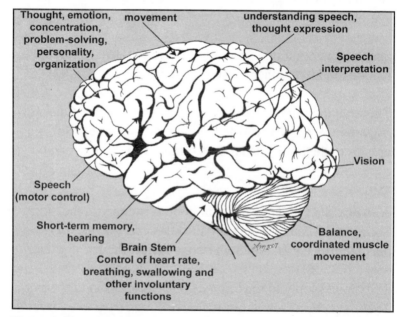

Figure 1. Functional locations of the brain

How is stroke diagnosed?

Strokes are often evaluated in an emergent setting (e.g., a hospital emergency room). Tests include blood samples to rule out blood abnormalities such as low blood sugar which can sometimes mimic stroke symptoms, as well as imaging of the brain with either a *CT (computerized tomography) scan* or *MRI (magnetic resonance imaging) scan*. A CT scan is very useful at detecting hemorrhagic strokes but may be normal in an ischemic stroke, particularly if stroke is mild, or if performed within a few hours after the onset of symptoms. An MRI will virtually always show the signs of a stroke if performed within a few days of the stroke onset. However, an MRI is more time-consuming, more expensive and some patients cannot have MRI's due to claustrophobia or having metal, such as pacemakers, in their bodies.

What is a TIA?

TIA stands for *transient ischemic attack*. A TIA is essentially a stroke in which symptoms resolve entirely within 24 hours. Some refer to TIA's as "mini-strokes".

What is the treatment of stroke?

The only treatment shown to be effective for the immediate treatment of ischemic stroke is the clot-busting medicine known as *tissue plasminogen activator (tPA)*. If given within 3 hours of the onset of symptoms, tPA has been shown to improve the chance of near-complete recovery from an ischemic stroke by about 30%. tPA cannot be given in the setting of a hemorrhagic stroke, which is why CT scan is usually obtained emergently to rule out hemorrhage. tPA treatment carries some risk and can actually cause hemorrhage into the brain in about 6% of treated patients.

Most stroke care is supportive, which means monitoring for other medical illnesses that may develop, such as infections, and starting rehabilitation with physical therapy, occupational therapy and speech therapy.

How is stroke prevented?

The risk factors for ischemic stroke are very similar to coronary heart disease. Treatment of high blood pressure, high cholesterol, diabetes, smoking cessation, healthy diet and regular exercise has been shown to prevent recurrent stroke.

Also, medicines that decrease the stickiness of platelets in the bloodstream such as aspirin, *clopidogrel (Plavix)* and *aspirin/dipyrridamole (Aggrenox)* can be used to prevent stroke. A more potent blood thinner, *warfarin (coumadin)*, is often used if the stroke was thought to have been caused by a blood clot that originated in the heart and migrated to the brain.

Procedures to open up partially blocked arteries, particularly the carotid arteries in the neck, can also help prevent recurrent strokes. Preventing recurrent hemorrhagic stroke depends on the cause of the initial hemorrhage. Hemorrhage can be due to various causes such as extreme high blood pressure, vascular anomalies such as aneurysms or blood-clotting deficiencies.

What is dementia?

Dementia, simply put, means that a patient has developed impairment in memory and some other area of cognition (such as language or decision-making) severe enough to affect his or her daily functioning. Any disease that afflicts the brain can technically cause dementia. However, the most common cause of dementia is Alzheimer's disease and the terms are sometimes used interchangeably. About 4 million people in the United States are thought to have Alzheimer's disease. The second-most common cause of dementia is probably *multiple strokes*, commonly referred to as *multi-infarct dementia* or *vascular dementia*.

What is Alzheimer's disease?

Alzheimer's disease is a slowly progressive disorder of the brain that usually starts with "short-term" memory loss but eventually causes *language problems*, *impaired judgment*, *visuoperceptual difficulties* and *personality changes*. The cause of Alzheimer's disease is not completely known, but most researchers believe that a build-up of a protein in the brain called *amyloid beta* may be the main problem. This protein forms clumps called *amyloid plaques* which can be seen on an autopsy of the brain of a person who dies with Alzheimer's disease.

How is Alzheimer's disease diagnosed in a living patient?

The diagnosis of Alzheimer's disease is never 100% certain in a patient still alive. However, if the patient has typical symptoms, and other conditions that affect memory (such as multiple strokes, medication problems, depression) have been ruled out, then the diagnosis can be over 90% certain.

How do I know if my forgetfulness is Alzheimer's or not?

If you are worried about forgetfulness, chances are it is not Alzheimer's disease. Our brains were simply not made to remember everything that happens to us in the course of the day, particularly in our current culture of excess information. Because of the nature of the memory impairment, many Alzheimer's patients are not even aware of their memory problems. There's a saying, "If you remember you forgot, that's o.k.; if you forget that you forgot, that's not." Since serious memory problems are often more noticeable to others than to yourself, ask your family or friends if they have been concerned about your memory.

How is Alzheimer's disease treated?

Four medications have been shown to temporarily stabilize the progression of Alzheimer's symptoms. Three of these medicines work on boosting a chemical in the brain called *acetylcholine* and are called *donepezil (Aricept)*, *galantamine (Razadyne)* and *rivastigmine (Exelon)*. These three are approved for the mild to moderate stages of Alzheimer's disease. A fourth medicine, *memantine (Namenda)*, works on the chemical *glutamate* and is approved for the moderate to severe stages of Alzheimer's disease. These medicines can stabilize symptoms for anywhere from 3 months to a year, but ultimately Alzheimer's disease continues to progress. Treatment of behavioral problems and depression and education of caregivers is another important aspect of Alzheimer's treatment.

What can I do to prevent Alzheimer's disease?

Unfortunately, many enterprising individuals have taken advantage of the public's fear of Alzheimer's disease by writing books on prevention or pushing vitamin and herbal supplements, all for the benefit of their own pocketbook. However, to date, nothing is clearly scientifically proven to prevent Alzheimer's disease.

Preliminary evidence does seem to indicate that a healthy diet with plenty of antioxidants (found in colorful fruits and vegetables) and lean meats (particularly fish) may lower the risk of Alzheimer's disease. Also, people who remain physically and mentally active late in life seem to have a lower rate of Alzheimer's disease.

But Alzheimer's disease probably starts years before it is actually diagnosed, and the first symptoms may actually be a decline in activity levels.

In this author's opinion, Alzheimer's disease is not "a use or lose it" disease. Alzheimer's is a disease like many other diseases, such as muscular dystrophy, and not too many would tell a child with muscular dystrophy he has to use his legs or he'll lose them. Nonetheless, just as regular exercise in muscular dystrophy may help preserve some strength, keeping cognitively active may help stave off some of the effects of Alzheimer's disease.

What is my risk of Alzheimer's disease?

The two biggest risk factors for Alzheimer's disease are clearly *aging* and a *family history* of Alzheimer's. On average, about 8 percent of the population is diagnosed with Alzheimer's disease at age 75. By age 95, up to 30 to 40 percent of individuals may have Alzheimer's disease. If you have one first-degree family member (meaning parent or sibling) diagnosed with Alzheimer's, your risk roughly doubles, such that you would have a 16-percent chance of Alzheimer's by age 75. If you have two first-degree family members with Alzheimer's, then your risk would about triple to 24 percent by age 75.

What is Parkinson's disease?

Somewhat like Alzheimer's disease, *Parkinson's disease* is another degenerative condition affecting the brain and is increasingly common as we age. Approximately 1 million people in the United States have Parkinson's disease.

Parkinson's disease afflicts mostly the motor systems of the brain, leading to problems such as *tremors*, a *slowing down and stiffness of movements* and *walking problems*. In

49

Parkinson's disease, a part of the brain called the ***substantia nigra*** is losing nerve cells at a faster rate than normal. This supplies the chemical ***dopamine*** to other areas of the brain. However, just as Alzheimer's is only one cause of dementia, Parkinson's disease is only one cause of "Parkinsonism." Many other conditions such as ***multiple stroke***, ***medication effects*** and ***hydrocephalus*** (sometimes called ***"water on the brain"***) can mimic Parkinson's disease symptoms.

How is Parkinson's disease treated?

A medication called ***L-dopa*** that directly replaces dopamine can sometimes provide dramatic relief of symptoms of Parkinson's disease. L-dopa usually comes combined with other medications to minimize side effects and prolong the action. These medicines are known as ***carbidopa/levodopa (sinemet) and carbidopa/levodopa/entacapone (stalevo)***. However, long-term use of L-dopa is thought to be associated with a problem called ***dyskinesias***, in which patients develop a restless sensation with writhing movements of the extremities. Therefore, in younger patients, the use of L-dopa is delayed as long as possible.

Some other common medications used to treat Parkinson's disease mimic dopamine and are called ***pramipexole (Mirapex)*** and ***ropinirole (Requip)***. Several other medications that prevent the breakdown of dopamine or act on other chemical systems in the brain are also somewhat beneficial in Parkinson's disease.

Physical therapy and speech therapy can also be very helpful for some patients.

Can someone die because of Parkinson's disease or Alzheimer's disease?

No one really dies directly because of either Parkinson's or

Alzheimer's disease. Although Parkinson's disease is more treatable than Alzheimer's, if someone lives long enough with either disease, they will ultimately progress to the point that mobility and swallowing problems can develop. When this occurs, the risk of pneumonia, other infections and blood clots increases dramatically and is the usual cause of death. Some overlap exists in the symptoms of Parkinson's disease and Alzheimer's disease and one condition referred to as *Lewy Body Disease* can clearly mimic both disorders.

Are there any cures for Alzheimer's disease or Parkinson's disease on the horizon?

There probably are not any cures in the immediate future. However, since Parkinson's disease affects a more restricted area of the brain, *implanting deep-brain stimulators* in certain areas has already shown substantial benefits, and *stem cell transplants* or nerve growth injections into similar areas look promising. *Medications that block or clear the beta-amyloid aggregation* in Alzheimer's disease seem the most promising. Also, both diseases may eventually be diagnosed before symptoms start with specialized brain scans called **PET** or *SPECT scans* that measure amyloid beta build-up or dopamine deficiency.

Should I be concerned about any other brain conditions?

Another common problem in the elderly is *drug-induced side effects*. The cognitive problems and motor symptoms already described can also be caused by medications. Anyone developing these symptoms who is on multiple medications should always check the possibility of reducing the dose or stopping any non-essential medications with their prescribing physician.

Many medications (including the over-the-counter medicine

benadryl) have an *"anticholinergic effect"* which can impair short-term memory.

Some medicines such as *neuroleptics* and *anti-nausea medicines* can cause Parkinsonism, and many medicines can cause tremors.

Also, diagnoses such as Parkinson's disease and Alzheimer's disease can be very difficult to diagnose in someone who has multiple health problems. For example, in a particular patient, *walking problems* may be caused by severe *arthritis*, *tremors* as a *medication effect* and concentration or memory problems from being in *chronic pain* or *sleep-deprived*.

A related point is that people do not require less sleep as they age but actually more because sleep becomes more fragmented. *Inadequate sleep* is a common cause of a decline in the quality of life.

What else can I do to keep my brain healthy?

Taking care of your general health is essential. After all, other organs such as the heart, lungs, kidney and liver all exist to provide the right blood flow and nutrients to the brain. A healthy diet and exercise have already been mentioned. Ideally, exercise should occur at least 30 to 60 minutes most days of the week.

Also, *"moderate" alcohol consumption* may also be beneficial for the brain. Moderate is defined as no more than two drinks a day for men and one drink a day for women. However, check with your physician before drinking alcohol if you are on any prescription drugs.

There is also increasing evidence that chronic worry and anxiety are unhealthy for the brain. **So most important of**

all is to try and enjoy life. Even with all the seemingly bad things that can happen to our brain, many people retain their cognitive abilities well into their 90's. Many people are happier later in their lives than they ever were when they were younger.

Summary
To summarize, keeping the brain healthy in aging is complicated, with no easy answer. Nonetheless, to paraphrase, **what's good for the body is good for the brain**. Eat plenty of fruits and vegetables and low-fat meats, exercise regularly, obtain adequate sleep, drink alcohol in moderation and enjoy life.

How to Respond to Emergencies
When Every Second Counts
Lori Christensen, RN

I am having chest pain: Could it be a heart attack?

A *heart attack* happens when your heart is not receiving the oxygen it needs. The signs and symptoms of a heart attack can be any of the following:

- Pressure or crushing pain in the chest that could feel like an elephant sitting on your chest.
- Radiation of pain that could go to the left arm, jaw or back.
- Sweating, nausea and vomiting.
- Shortness of breath with or without the chest pain.

Assess your pain. Do you have the pain with activity or at rest? How long does the pain last? What symptoms do you have? What does relieve the pain? **If you are having these symptoms, you need to seek help immediately by calling 9-1-1. Calling 9-1-1 is the fastest way to get medical attention.** Driving yourself to the hospital should not be an option unless there are absolutely no other options. Time is the key factor if you think you are having a heart attack. **Never hesitate to seek medical help if you think you are having a heart attack. It is better to be safe than sorry.**

What is sublingual nitroglycerin?

Nitroglycerin – or "nitro" – is a medicine that relaxes the blood vessels of the heart thereby improving blood flow and oxygen to part of your heart muscles. You are to use the nitro if you experience sudden chest pain. Here are some simple steps for the use of nitro:

- Lie down or sit when taking nitro.
- Place one tablet under your tongue and leave it there until it dissolves.
- If you are still having the chest pain after 5 minutes of taking your first nitro, call 9-1-1 immediately.
- Take another nitro at this point; you can take up to 3 doses total 5 minutes apart.
- If you are using the nitro spray instead of the tablets, you do one spray under the tongue. The same steps apply for the spray as for the tablets.

The side effects of nitro include dizziness, warm or flushed feeling, headache, lightheadedness and a temporary burning sensation under the tongue. ***DO NOT*** take nitro if you take a medicine for erectile dysfunction such as Viagra, Levitra, or Cialis. This can cause a life-threatening drop in your blood pressure and can lead to serious complications. A good tablet should taste bitter and cause a slight sting when you put it underneath your tongue. Always make sure you check the expiration date on your bottle as pills that are expired will not be as effective. And lastly, no matter what happens, be sure to notify your physician to make them aware of what happened.

Learning CPR: The basics

CPR stands for ***cardiopulmonary resuscitation***. CPR provides blood supply and oxygen to the vital organs of a person who loses pulse or quits breathing. Here are some pointers on how to perform CPR. Taking a certified CPR class would also be ***VERY*** beneficial and is highly recommended.

If you are in a situation where CPR needs to be initiated, here are some pointers:

- **Check for responsiveness.** Check to see if the

person responds by shaking and loudly asking "Are you ok?"

- **Call 9-1-1 if there is no response.** If there are people around you, yell for them to call 9-1-1. If you are alone, leave the person to call 9-1-1.
- **Place the person on his/her back.**
- **Open the airway.** This is done by lifting the chin up with two fingers and at the same time pushing down on the forehead with your other hand.
- **Look, listen, and feel for breathing.** Place your ear by the person's nose, mouth and feel for the breath on your face and look to the chest for movement.
- **If the person is not breathing:** You need to put your mouth tightly over the person's mouth, pinch the nose closed, keep the person's head in the same position as above and give two full slow breaths. If the chest doesn't rise, be sure that your mouth is completely covering the person's mouth.
- **Look for signs of circulation** by checking the person to see if there is movement or breathing. If you know how to check a pulse, this is the time to do it. If neither of those is present, you need to begin chest compressions.
    - Chest compressions are done by placing the heel of one hand right between the nipples and placing the heel of your other hand on top of the first hand and interlocking your fingers.
    - Position yourself directly over the person. You should be looking directly down at your hands if you are in the correct position.
    - Give 30 compressions total that should be fast and about two inches into the chest.
    - After you give the compressions, you need to give two more slow, full breaths and continue this cycle of 30 compressions and 2 breaths for about 1 minute and then re-check for signs

of movement, coughing or breathing.

- o If the person is still not breathing, keep doing this cycle until help arrives.
- o If the person does start to breathe again, make sure you monitor them for breathing and movement.

These pointers should help you if you are ever in a situation that would require you to use CPR. Training in CPR to better familiarize yourself in these steps is a great idea because CPR can be life-saving!

Abdominal Pain: Should I wait?

Abdominal pain is a pain you can feel in between your lower chest and your groin. This pain can range from mild to severe in intensity. Sometimes severe abdominal pain can be caused from a mild condition such as gas. The most important thing to do is monitor your symptoms.

For mild pains, try to avoid solid food for a couple of hours and sip on water or other clear fluids (i.e., broth, 7-Up, Jello, etc.)

If the pain is high in your abdomen and feels like your food is just "sitting there," try an antacid such as Rolaids.

If you experience sudden, sharp abdominal pain, you need to seek medical attention right away. Other associated symptoms you could have with the abdominal pain are vomiting blood, dark and tarry stools, or your abdomen could feel hard and painful to the touch.

Serious causes of abdominal pain could be an *aortic dissection*, *kidney stones*, *appendicitis*, and *gallstones,* all which require medical attention immediately. If you are unsure as to what is causing your abdominal pain, call your doctor. Symptoms such as *diarrhea* or *bloating* or *vomiting* usually only last a few days. If these symptoms don't resolve in a few days, be sure to call your doctor and make him/her aware of what is going on and how long it's been happening.

Some ways to prevent abdominal pain include eating small frequent meals that are high in fiber, avoiding foods that cause gas, and drinking plenty of water daily. If you are unsure of what to do, call your doctor for guidance.

Fainting spells: What to do next . . .

Fainting (also sometimes referred to as *syncope*) is a temporary loss of consciousness due to a lack of blood supply to your brain. The episode is usually brief, and some people get dizzy or lightheaded or feel weak or nauseated before the fainting happens. Fainting can be related to several things, such as low blood sugar, standing in one place too long, severe dehydration (lack of fluids in your body), a *rhythm disturbance* in the heart or *seizures*.

If you are alone and you faint, call your doctor as soon as you regain consciousness to get an appointment as soon as possible. If you have fainted before and you know the situations that cause you to faint, try to avoid them. Get up from a lying or sitting position slowly and avoid sudden changes in your posture. If you are fainting continually, you need to seek medical attention right away to be evaluated. Medications for anxiety, allergies, and high blood pressure can also be a cause of fainting because they drop your blood pressure. Fainting is a symptom, not a disease, and can be treated.

Chest pain or heartburn: How do I know?

Do you know how to tell the difference if you are actually

having **chest pain** or if it is just **heartburn**? Heartburn produces a burning sensation in your chest that can radiate to your neck. It can also leave a sour taste in your mouth after lying down. Heartburn is caused by stomach acid flowing back into your esophagus. Heartburn can feel similar to the symptoms you can have with chest pain. However, you usually will not notice a sudden pressure or crushing pain in the center of your chest that lasts more than a few minutes. Pain from heartburn feels more like a burning.

Chest pain usually produces pain that can spread to the back, neck, jaw, arms, or shoulders and can be accompanied by shortness of breath, sweating, nausea, or dizziness. While heartburn can definitely make you feel nauseous, you should not experience any shortness of breath or sweating or dizziness with the heartburn. Heartburn comes about mainly after you eat a big meal or lie down after eating a meal. Certain foods, such as caffeine products or alcohol, can increase the production of stomach acid.

When do you know to get help? If you just occasionally get heartburn, try using a medicine for acid control and take it about an hour before you eat a meal. For fast relief, try Rolaids, etc. If you have the burning sensation on a daily basis, call your doctor for further evaluation.

Heartburn is not an emergent problem, but *if the burning is associated with a crushing pain or tightening in the chest, shortness of breath, sweating, nausea, dizziness, or pain that radiates to your neck, arm, jaw, back or shoulders, seek medical attention right away.*

How does my emergency alert device work?

An *emergency alert device* helps you to stay independent in your home while help is only a push away. When you purchase an alert device, you give your doctor information about your emergency contact and essential medical information. Your emergency alert device can help if you suffer from a fall or from chest pain or any other emergency that disables you to where you can't get to a phone. All you have to do is press the button and help will be on the way. Make sure you keep your alert device on you and accessible. The last thing you need is to have an emergency and your alert device isn't even near you. If you think an emergency alert device is something you would be interested in, you could get it online (if applicable) or call your insurance company or speak with your doctor.

My heart feels like it's jumping out of my chest! Should I worry?

If you have ever experienced this feeling before it is called a *palpitation,* or a "skipped beat." A palpitation can be something that comes and goes every once in a while or it could be due to an *abnormal heart rhythm,* also called *arrhythmia*. Palpitations can also be caused by stress, anxiety, caffeine and alcohol consumption.

- Slow arrhythmias are slower than 60 beats per minute.
- Rapid arrhythmias are greater than 100 beats per minute.

So how do you know if it is something serious? Here are some tips:

- For a rapid arrhythmia, the palpitation may feel like your heart is pulsing in the neck or a fluttering, thumping, or pounding in the chest. It may also feel like a racing beat in the chest. You could also experience chest discomfort, weakness, fainting, and shortness of breath, confusion or dizziness. If you experience any of these symptoms, you need to get

61

help immediately.
- For slow arrhythmia, you could experience shortness of breath, lightheadedness, fatigue or even loss of consciousness. You need to seek help immediately.

If it is a palpitation that occurs occasionally, contact your physician to make him/her aware of what is happening. Your doctor might want to do an electrocardiogram (EKG) to make sure you aren't in an abnormal heart rhythm. The doctor might also want to order some blood work. Some of the electrolytes in your body, such as potassium, can cause abnormal heart rhythms if too low or too high. The doctor could also order a *Holter monitor* or possibly an event monitor to monitor your heart continuously. A Holter monitor is short-term, while an event monitor is kept on for one month. Palpitations can be relieved in many patients by reducing stress, stopping smoking, and reducing your intake of caffeine and alcohol. In some cases medications do need to be prescribed.

I am diabetic: What should I know if my blood sugar goes too high or too low?

Hypoglycemia, or *low blood sugar,* occurs when sugar levels in the blood are too low. It can happen if a diabetic individual doesn't eat enough food, takes too much insulin, does vigorous exercise without eating a snack beforehand, waits too long between meals or drinks excessive alcohol.
- During the early stages of a hypoglycemic episode, symptoms include sweating, tremor, hunger and anxiety.
- If left untreated, hypoglycemia can cause weakness, lethargy, lack of coordination, blurred vision or personality changes, confusion, unconsciousness and coma.
- Drinking one cup of sweetened juice or eating six to

eight hard candies can easily treat symptoms. Once the person's symptoms and blood glucose levels are under control, the person should eat cheese and crackers or drink a glass of milk to prevent symptoms from returning.

Hyperglycemia is what happens when your blood sugar becomes too high. Causes of hyperglycemia can include eating more than planned or exercising less than planned. Illnesses like a cold or flu can also cause hyperglycemia. Symptoms include a high blood sugar level, frequent urination and increased thirst.

If left untreated, this can cause *ketoacidosis,* or *diabetic coma* can occur. This develops when your body doesn't have enough insulin. Symptoms of ketoacidosis include shortness of breath, breath that smells fruity, a very dry mouth, nausea and vomiting. Ketoacidosis is life-threatening and requires immediate attention. Ketoacidosis is managed in the hospital where a patient receives insulin intravenously and is well hydrated with close monitoring of his or her electrolytes. The key to preventing hyperglycemia is to know the symptoms and to treat them when it happens before it can get worse.

I have a headache – what should I do?

Pain from a *headache* can be in only one part of the head or it could involve the whole head. The type of pain you can experience ranges from constant and dull or sudden and sharp. You can also experience other signs with your headache, such as nausea. There are three main types of headaches.

- *Migraine headaches* are throbbing and intense and involve one side of the head. You can be sensitive to light or noise. These headaches can last from hours to days.

- ***Tension headaches*** feel like a tightening on both sides of the head. These headaches are usually caused by stress or bad posture. These headaches can be frequent and last minutes to days.
- ***Cluster headaches*** are non-throbbing and mostly on one side of the head behind an eye. These headaches are usually due to increased blood flow to the blood vessels in the brain. They can last 30-45 minutes and occur over several days.

Contact your doctor if you have to take a pain reliever every day for your headache or if you have three or more headaches a week. Very few headaches that have serious underlying problems do not require immediate medical attention. **If you experience a headache with any other symptoms such as problems with vision or slurred speech, vomiting, loss of balance, shortness of breath, fever and/or stiff neck, you need to seek medical attention immediately.**

Sudden shortness of breath: What do I do?

Shortness of breath (sometimes called ***dyspnea)*** can be caused by abnormalities in different areas of the body. If it is severe and sudden it could be related to a problem requiring immediate attention. It doesn't matter if the shortness of breath is short or long in duration. If you notice the shortness of breath with rest or with activity, when lying down, or on exposure to allergens, you should seek help right away. If you experience sudden shortness of breath with any of the following symptoms, you should seek help immediately.

- Chest pain or discomfort or pain that radiates to your jaw or neck.
- Fluid weight gain (edema) of three pounds or more in one day.
- Yellow-, green-, or rusty-colored sputum (saliva).
- Blue discoloration of your lips or fingertips.

- Fainting, dizzy spells, or lightheadedness.
- Pain when taking a deep breath.
- Unusual fatigue that is sudden.

Sudden shortness of breath can be caused by lung problems such as a blood clot or asthma, heart problems such as heart failure, kidney or chronic liver problems, shock from extremely low blood pressure, fever, and increased pressure in the brain caused by trauma or stroke. The most important thing to do is to evaluate your symptoms. As above, if you experience sudden shortness of breath accompanied by any of the symptoms listed, you need to seek medical attention immediately.

Fever and chills: Is this an emergency?

Chills are an episode of shivering with paleness and a feeling of coldness. Chills are caused by rapid muscular contraction and relaxation and are the body's way to produce heat when your body thinks that you are cold. Chills often represent the onset of fever. Common causes of chills include:

- Colds
- Influenza
- Strep throat
- Viral gastroenteritis
- Bacterial gastroenteritis
- Urinary tract infections
- Pneumonia
- Meningitis

Fever is the body's natural response to a variety of conditions in the body. If the fever is 101.5 degrees Fahrenheit or lower with no other symptoms, no immediate attention is required. Just be sure to drink plenty of fluids and get plenty of rest. Using warm water (about 70 degrees Fahrenheit) is the best way to help reduce a fever. Cold water could be uncomfortable and may increase the fever because cold water can produce chills. Do not bundle up with blankets as this can cause the fever to rise. Call your doctor if:

- You have a significant cough, abdominal pain or burning or frequency in urination.
- There is stiffness in your neck, confusion, irritability, or sluggishness.
- Fever remains above 102 degrees Fahrenheit after two hours (if self-treatment doesn't work).
- The fever doesn't improve in 3 days or has lasted more than 5 days.

If any of the symptoms are severe, seek medical attention immediately. If you are unsure, call your doctor first for direction.

I am on diuretics (water pills) and have leg cramps: Is there a relationship?

Diuretics are medications that help stimulate the kidneys to produce more urine which flushes excess fluids and **electrolytes** (including potassium) from the body. Diuretics are used in a variety of conditions, such as heart failure or high blood pressure. If you are initiated on a diuretic, you will normally have lab work a couple of days after starting to monitor your electrolytes. If you are experiencing leg cramps after starting on a diuretic, it could possibly be in an **electrolyte imbalance**.

However, if the leg cramps were present before you started the diuretic, it would be a good idea to contact your doctor for further follow-up. Some diuretics are "potassium-sparing," which means that the potassium doesn't get flushed out of the body. This could cause **hyperkalemia** or a high blood potassium level. A high potassium level can cause muscle weakness, numbness and tingling, which could definitely show up in your legs.

If you start to develop these symptoms, contact the doctor who prescribed the medicine to let him/her know the symptoms you are having. Do not stop taking the medication unless directed to do so by your doctor. Your doctor will give you further instruction on what to do next.

If you develop any other symptoms such as severe low blood pressure, a fast or irregular heartbeat, severe dizziness or fainting, deafness or ringing in the ears, excessive thirst, weak pulse, or confusion, you need to seek help immediately.

Is it a stroke? What should I do?

A *stroke* is an interruption of the blood flow to the brain causing damage to brain tissue. A stroke can be caused by blood clots, high blood pressure, drug abuse, or head injury. Symptoms of a stroke are usually sudden and include:

- Numbness, tingling or decreased sensation
- Weakness or paralysis of side of face, arm, leg, or any part of the body
- Vision changes
- Slurred speech, inability to speak or difficulty with reading or writing
- Loss of coordination or balance
- Loss of memory
- Difficulties swallowing
- Drooling
- Mood changes
- Drowsiness or loss of consciousness
- Eyelid drooping or uncontrolled eye movements

If you experience any of these symptoms, call 9-1-1 immediately. A stroke is a medical emergency that requires immediate attention to save your life! Immediate treatment is the best treatment as time is a ***BIG*** factor in stroke treatment.

How long should I be on blood thinners after a stent is placed? What are the consequences if I go off of them earlier?

A *stent* is a metal mesh placed in the arteries of the heart to open blockages. A patient should be on a blood thinner which includes a combination of ***Plavix*** and aspirin for one month if he or she had a ***bare metal stent (non-medicated stent)***. If the patient has had a ***drug-eluting stent (medicated stent)***, then Plavix and aspirin are recommended for one year, then aspirin alone indefinitely.

If the patient is taken off or decides to go off the Plavix and aspirin, a blood clot could form on the stent and a heart attack or possibly death might occur.

After one year if there are no recurring problems or any other indication for the Plavix, it can be discontinued. The most important thing to do is take the Plavix as directed by your doctor.

If you have problems with taking the medication such as upset stomach or rash or itching, contact your doctor first. **DO NOT stop the medicine on your own.** Or if you have any questions in general, be sure to contact your doctor first. If a clot forms on the stents, symptoms of heart attack occur and you should seek immediate medical attention.

Tips to Reduce High Blood Pressure
Nidal Harb, MD, FACC, FACP

Over the past 25 years, there has been tremendous progress in the way we treat heart disease. This includes the development of new procedures and techniques to treat cardiovascular diseases.

Since 1919, *cardiovascular diseases* have been the number one killer in the United States contributing to the death of 40% of all Americans. Worldwide, more than half of the population suffers from complications of *atherosclerosis*, or hardening of the arteries.

What is hypertension?
Hypertension, or *high blood pressure*, is one of the most common cardiovascular diseases. It affects about 50,000,000 Americans. The prevalence of hypertension increases as we age. Nearly two-thirds of men and women in their 60's and 70's have high blood pressure.

Why is high blood pressure a serious health condition?
High blood pressure is a serious condition because it can cause target organ damage which affects the heart, the kidneys, the eyes, the brain and the blood vessels.

The impact of hypertension is taxing both in terms of cost and loss of life. The estimated direct and indirect cost is almost $50 billion.

High blood pressure is frequently called the silent killer since many patients are not aware of the problem. Even for those who are aware of the problem, only a small percentage has good blood pressure control.

What is a "normal" blood pressure reading?

A *normal blood pressure* refers to a blood pressure of less than 120/80 mmHg. However, readings of above or equal 140/90 mmHg are considered *high blood pressure*. In patients with diabetes, renal failure, or heart failure we tend to consider the blood pressure to be elevated if it is above 125/80 mmHg.

What are the causes of hypertension?

In more than 90% of the people with hypertension there was no obvious cause for this condition. *Genetic factors* and *family history* may play a major role. The condition is most commonly seen in middle-age and elderly patients because of the *rigidity of the arteries associated with age*. High blood pressure is more commonly initially seen with men; however, later on women will catch up. It is also seen with patients who are *overweight* or *drink a large amount of alcohol*.

In the minority of cases, the underlying cause of high blood pressure is identified *as blockage in the arteries of the kidneys*, or kidney disease itself. Other possibilities are *hormonal disorders*, such as *Cushing syndrome* or *hyperaldosteronism* associated with a high blood level of cortisol or aldosterone respectively. Both cortisol and aldosterone can lead to sodium and water retention and eventually high blood pressure. Sometimes *medications* like steroids or oral contraceptives may also cause hypertension. When the cause of hypertension can be identified this is called *secondary hypertension*.

One of the most important causes of secondary hypertension is *sleep apnea*, which is more commonly seen with patients with hypertension and associated with several adverse conditions, including irregular heartbeat or heart failure. The symptoms of sleep apnea include heavy snoring, increased day sleepiness, and fatigue.

There is also a condition called *"white-coat" hypertension* where the blood pressure is always elevated at the doctor's office. In order to rule out this condition, we commonly ask patients to monitor their blood pressure outside the office.

Is there a "cure" for hypertension?

Hypertension usually cannot be cured; however, it can be controlled with appropriate treatment, which initially involves lifestyle modifications and, if necessary, using different medications, which will be discussed in detail later in this chapter.

In most cases, these measures can control the high blood pressure and reduce the risk of complications. These measures usually need to be maintained indefinitely, although in some cases we may be able to cut down on the number of medications. In the cases of secondary hypertension, we may be able to cure the disease if the underlying cause is treated.

BLOOD PRESSURE MEASUREMENT TECHNIQUES

METHOD	NOTES
In-office	Two readings, 5 minutes apart, sitting in chair. Confirm elevated reading in contralateral arm.
Ambulatory BP monitoring	Indicated for evaluation of "white coat hypertension." Absence of 10-20 percent BP decrease during sleep may indicate increased CVD risk.
Patient self-check	Provides information on response to therapy. May help improve adherence to therapy and is useful for evaluating "white coat hypertension".

CLASSIFICATION OF BLOOD PRESSURE (BP)

Category	SBP mmHg		DBP mmHg
Normal	<120	and	<80
Prehypertension	120-139	or	80-89
Hypertension, stage I	140-159	or	90-99
Hypertension, stage 2	≥160	or	≥100

SBP = Systolic blood pressure
DBP = Diastolic blood pressure

What lifestyle modifications are helpful in treating hypertension?

- DASH eating plan
- dietary sodium restriction
- aerobic physical activity
- limited, if any, consumption of alcohol
- weight reduction

Principles of lifestyle modification

Encourage healthy lifestyles for all individuals. Prescribe lifestyle modifications for all patients with prehypertension and hypertension.

LIFESTYLE MODIFICATION RECOMMENDATIONS

Modification	Recommendation	Avg SBP Reduction [†]
Weight reduction	**Maintain normal body weight (body mass index 18.5-24.9 kg/m^2)**	**5-20 mmHg/10 kg**
DASH eating plan	**Adopt a diet rich in fruits, vegetables, and low fat dairy products with reduced content of saturated and total fat.**	**8-14 mmHg**
Dietary sodium reduction	**Reduce dietary sodium intake to $\leq$ 100 mmol per day (2.4 g sodium or 6 g sodium chloride)**	**2-8 mmHg**
Aerobic physical activity	**Regular aerobic physical activity (e.g. brisk walking) at least 30 minutes per day, most days of the week)**	**4-9 mmHg**
Moderation of alcohol consumption	**Men: Limit to $\leq$2 drinks* per day. Women and lighter weight persons: Limit to $\leq$1 drink* per day**	**2-4 mmHg**

* 1 drink = ½ oz or 15 mL ethanol (e.g. 12 oz beer, 5 oz wine, 1.5 oz 80-proof whiskey).

[†] **Effects are dose and time dependent**

What types of medications are available to treat hypertension?

Over the past 50 years, there has been a significant drop in the incidence of heart attacks and strokes. One of the main reasons for this drop is the development of newer medications to treat high blood pressure. Nowadays, there are more than 100 different medications which could be used to treat this ailment. There is also a combination of different drugs which also could be utilized.

The most commonly used drugs are:
- *Diuretic drugs*
- *Beta-blockers*
- *Calcium channel blockers*
- *ACE inhibitors*
- *Alpha blockers*
- *Angiotensin II blockers (ARBs)*
- *Centrally acting drugs*
- *Other antihypertensive medications*

Beta-blockers, ACE inhibitors, ARBs and calcium channel blockers, in addition to diuretics, are the most commonly used medications. Less frequently used are centrally acting drugs and alpha-blockers, in addition to other drugs, including hydralazine and minoxidil.

Most **antihypertensive medications** reduce high blood pressure by relaxing the vessel wall, thus increasing the diameter of the vessel. Others may reduce the force with which the heart pumps the blood. **Diuretics** will cause increased urine outputs, which will result in reduced volume of blood present in the circulation. This chapter will provide useful information about high blood pressure medications, as well as potential alternatives. Certainly, this book is not intended to tell you which, if any, medication is best for you, since this only can be determined by your physician after appropriate evaluation.

These medications usually have two names. One is called brand name, which may differ from one company to another depending on the pharmaceutical manufacturer. They all, however, share the same generic name, which refers to all medications with the same chemical structure. In the USA, due to FDA regulations, the brand and generic names should be equal in effectiveness and safety. Sometimes, the tablets may differ in size or color due to the inactive substance, which is usually added to the medications. Your physician may allow the use of generic medications; however, keep in mind that not all brand names can be obtained generically because of the patent protection law in the USA.

Once medication is taken, it is absorbed in the stomach or gut and then processed in the liver, eventually being eliminated from the body either through the kidney or through the liver. In order to obtain a certain level of medication in the body, the drug has to be taken on a certain schedule depending on the medications used. Some of those medications have a special delivery system, which makes them long-acting.

On many occasions, each medicine has different indications. Your doctor will individualize treatment based on your specific problems. Each medication may be used for several different medical problems.

Angiotensin converting enzyme inhibitors, or ACEI, is a group of medications that dilate the arteries and decrease the resistance to the flow of blood being pumped from the heart. The result is lowering of the blood pressure and easier pumping of the heart. This group includes medications like captopril, enalapril and lisinopril, among others. The side effects may include a rash, persistent dry cough and swelling of the skin. They also can elevate the potassium blood level and, therefore, occasional blood tests should be done to check for potassium level and kidney function. ACEI are utilized to treat high blood pressure and in patients with congestive heart failure. They are also given to patients with diabetes as they delay deterioration of kidney function.

The second group includes ***angiotensin receptive blockers***, or ARB. This includes medications like losartan, irbesartan, and valsartan, among others. They also dilate the arteries and decrease the resistance to the flow of blood being pumped from the heart. Blood tests should also be done to check for potassium and kidney function. ARB are utilized to treat high blood pressure and in patients with congestive heart failure. They are also given to patients with diabetes as they delay deterioration of kidney function.

The third group includes ***diuretics***, like furosemide and hydrochlorothiazide, among others. These medications will increase the urine output, thus decreasing the intravascular volume and reduce excess fluid in the body. This group of medications may lower the potassium level and, therefore, periodic testing should be done. Diuretics are given to patients with heart failure, high blood pressure or fluid overload.

The fourth group is called ***beta-blockers***, which include metoprolol, atenolol and propranolol, among others. This group will slow the heart beat, decrease the blood pressure and reduce the contraction strength of the heart muscle. These medications can slow the heart rate and can result in fatigue. Special precautions should be given for patients with asthma or those who have a slow heart rate. Beta-blockers can also cause impotence. These medications are effective in the treatment of angina, high blood pressure and heart failure. Also, they are very important in the treatment of patients who have experienced a heart attack and can reduce electrical disturbances in the heart.

The fifth group includes *calcium channel blockers*, such as verapamil, diltiazem, amlodipine and nifedipine. This group reduces the ability of calcium to enter the muscle of the heart and blood vessels, which will result in reduction of the heart rate, lowering of the squeezing strength of the heart muscle and dilatation of the blood vessel, thus lowering blood pressure. Calcium channel blockers can cause dizziness, constipation and lower extremity swelling. They are effective medications to treat angina and hypertension and some electrical disturbances in the heart.

The sixth group is called the *centrally acting agents*. These medications affect control centers in the brain that decrease blood pressure. Medications include methyldopa and clonidine, among others. Specific side effects include dry mouth, dizziness and drowsiness. Precautions should be given to avoid sudden blood pressure drop and dizziness by avoiding a sudden change in position. These medications are primarily used to treat high blood pressure.

The seventh group is called direct acting *vasodilators*, such as hydralazine and minoxidil. These medications cause the muscle in the walls of the blood vessels to relax. Specific side effects may include lupus syndrome and also the need to stand slowly from a lying position to avoid sudden blood pressure drop and dizziness. These medications are primarily used to treat high blood pressure.

The eighth group of medications includes *peripherally acting agents*, such as doxazosin and terazosin, among others. These medications exert their effect on the nerves of the body that are involved in blood pressure regulation. Similar precautions should be taken with regard to the sudden change in the position, which could result in a blood pressure drop and dizziness. These medications are primarily used to treat high blood pressure.

Do medications for high blood pressure react with grapefruit juice?

Over the past 15 years, there has been a great deal of research dealing with the mechanism and consequences of drug interaction with *grapefruit juice.* Several hundred publications have appeared in the scientific literature.

The medications will eventually be metabolized in the gastrointestinal system. Grapefruit juice contains a number of natural substances which may inhibit the metabolism of the medications and thus may increase the level of the medications in the blood.

Exposure to grapefruit juice requires about 48 to 72 hours for its effect to completely dissipate. Many times the exposure could result in clinically insignificant change in the medication levels. This interaction is only possible when the drug is given by mouth. Intravenous administrations will not interact with the grapefruit juice.

The magnitude of a drug interaction is different from drug to drug even if they were in the same class. For example, the lipid-lowering medications lovastatin and simvastatin will significantly interact with grapefruit juice, whereas others like pravastatin and fluvastatin have minimal interaction, if any. Individual variability is also a problem since it is unpredictable. The drug interaction with grapefruit juice usually will occur after a single exposure, for example, to a single 8-ounce glass. If the grapefruit juice is taken repeatedly, there is evidence to show that it will worsen the problem.

MEDICATION INTERACTION WITH GRAPEFRUIT JUICE

MEDICATION	MAGNITUDE OF INTERACTION		
	Large	*Moderate*	*Small or negligible*
Calcium Channel Antagonists		Felodipine Nicardipine Nifedipine Nimodipine Nisoldipine Isradipine	Amlodipine Diltiazem Verapamil
HMG-CoA reductase inhibitors (statins)	Lovastatin Simvastatin	Atorvastatin Cerivastatin	Fluvastatin Pravastatin
Immunosup-pressants		Cyclosporine Tacrolimus Sirolimus	
Sedative-hypnotic and anxiolytic agents	Buspirone	Triazolam Midazolam Diazepam Zaleplon	Alprazolam Clonazepam Zolpidem Temazepam Lorazepam
Other psychotropic agents		Carbamazepine Trazodone Nefazodone Quetiapine	SSRI antidepressants Clozapine Haloperidol
Antihistamines	Terfenadine Astemizole	Loratadine	Fexofenadine Cetirizine Diphenhydramine
Human immuno-deficiency virus protease inhibitors		Saquinavir Ritonavir Nelfinavir Amprenavir	Indinavir
Hormones		Ethinyl estradiol Methyl-prednisolone	Prednisone Prednisolone
Other medications	Amiodarone	Sildenafil Cisapride	Clarithromycin Erythromycin Quinidine Omeprazole

This list is not comprehensive and does not represent an endorsement of any product listed.

It is likely that although some drugs are affected by the interaction with grapefruit juice, most medications are not. There is always an alternative medication, which could be used with each drug class that allows appropriate treatments to proceed safely. *(See page 79 for summary of known and anticipated drug interactions with grapefruit juice.)*

In conclusion, engaging in lifestyle modifications and paying close attention to appropriate use of medications can help reduce high blood pressure. It is imperative that patients with hypertension follow up closely with their health care providers to monitor the effectiveness and safety of their medical treatment.

Diabetes Care: What You Need to Know
Danita Harrison, ARN, CDE

Diabetes is a very common disease that most likely either you have or you know someone who has it. Diabetes can be challenging to live with since it affects our lives on a daily basis. However, it is essential that you learn to live with diabetes, for if you take control of this disease and not let it control you, you can live a long, healthy life.

What is diabetes?

Diabetes is a condition that prevents your body from properly using *glucose (sugar)* for energy. Ideally, if our bodies are working properly, the amount of energy that is needed is provided by a balance of glucose and *insulin*. Insulin is produced by the *pancreas* in the beta cells. The pancreas is located by the stomach in the abdomen. Glucose comes from the food that is eaten, primarily food that contains carbohydrates.

What type of diabetes do I have?

There are several types of diabetes, but Type 1 and Type 2 will be addressed here.

Type 1 diabetes occurs when the beta cells located in the pancreas quit producing insulin. People with Type 1 diabetes must take insulin to stay alive. This type of diabetes is less common and often occurs when a person is young and thin.

The most common form of diabetes is *Type 2 diabetes*. Over time, the pancreas is not able to produce enough insulin to keep up with the body's needs. The body also has difficult time "allowing" insulin into the cell to work correctly in order to use sugar as energy in the body. Type 2 diabetes can be treated with medication, which may be oral or by injection, and/or insulin.

I have been told I have "pre-diabetes" – should I be concerned?

Yes, consider *"pre-diabetes"* a warning to adopt a better lifestyle immediately! A person without diabetes will normally have a fasting blood sugar under 100, or 2 hours after eating, under 140. Pre-diabetes occurs when a fasting blood sugar ranges between 100-125 or, after drinking 75 grams of glucose, having a blood sugar range of 140-199. These blood sugar ranges are not normal since diabetes is diagnosed one of 3 ways:

1. Symptoms of diabetes such as thirst, hunger, frequent urination or weight loss and a blood sugar at any time of over 200.
2. After fasting for at least 8 hours, with a blood sugar over 126.
3. A lab test of drinking 75 grams of glucose, with a blood sugar over 200 two hours later.

While a person with "pre-diabetes" has not been diagnosed yet with diabetes, the risk for cardiovascular disease such as heart attack, stroke and development of diabetes is quite high. A person with "pre-diabetes" should be monitored for the development of diabetes every year. The best thing you can do for your health with the pre-diabetes diagnosis is manage your weight and exercise daily!

What are the symptoms of diabetes?

Diabetes can go undiagnosed as a person ages, since the symptoms are often absent in the older adult. Therefore, many people are diagnosed at the time other illnesses are occurring. Symptoms of diabetes can include frequent thirst, urination, hunger and weight loss. However, because many adults do not notice signs of diabetes, they are not diagnosed until a routine lab test has been done.

After the age of 45, people should be screened for diabetes if they are overweight or have other risk factors such as high blood pressure, high cholesterol, gave birth to a baby over 9 pounds, or have relatives with diabetes, heart or blood vessel problems. The rate of diabetes is higher in the Asian American, African American, Hispanic, male Japanese, and Native American compared to Caucasian.

Why do I have to test my blood sugars at home?

Testing *blood sugars* at home is now easy and quick to do. If you have diabetes you should test your blood sugars at home. *Remember, you have to manage your blood sugars!* Self glucose monitoring helps give immediate glucose readings that can help you manage diabetes. By knowing your glucose readings, you receive immediate feedback on your current blood sugar, which can help in reaching your blood sugar goal, determine how your medication is working, help in treating low blood sugars and determine your blood sugar response to certain foods and activity. It is important to test your blood sugars on a regular basis, at a variety of times, including before and after meals! Blood sugar monitoring is important and needs to be done daily by those using insulin. Write down your blood sugar readings and take your records to every medical visit. Most insurance plans provide coverage for the meter and strips to test at home. Testing blood sugars at home requires one small drop of blood and less than one minute to obtain a reading, a small investment of your time which can yield significant benefits to your health and well-being.

What is an A1c (A one C) test?

An *A1c* is a blood test that shows the average blood sugar

for the past 2 to 3 months. This number is reflective of your blood sugar readings over time, including fasting, after eating and even sleeping!

A1c%	Average plasma glucose
6	135
7	170
8	205
9	240
10	275
11	310
12	345

(From 2007 ADA Clinical Practice Guidelines)

In general, your A1c should be below 7%, but do not ignore the fact people without diabetes have A1c values under 6%. Your A1c test should be completed at least twice a year if you have diabetes, even if it is under control! Having good A1c values or good diabetes control can help reduce your risk of eye, heart, kidney and nerve damage. So, in general, the lower your A1c value is, the better, but it should not be at the expense of having multiple low blood sugars.

How do I treat diabetes?

A lifestyle of keeping weight down and daily exercise, such as walking, is required to help maintain your diabetes health. Some people might need diabetes medications, as well. Diabetes tends to be a progressive disease and most people eventually will require medication to treat it. There are many medications now available for the treatment of diabetes. Each type of medication may work in a variety of different ways; therefore, more than one type of medication might be prescribed for the treatment of diabetes.

This list does not include all diabetes medications, nor does it list all of the possible side effects of each.

Oral agents

Sulfonylurea class: Some examples are *glyburide*, *glipizide* and *glimepiride*. These medications stimulate insulin to be produced from the pancreatic cells. Sulfonylureas tend to be lower cost and are generally taken 1 to 2 times a day. These medications can cause low blood sugar, so they should be taken at the same time every day, before eating. These drugs are absorbed more rapidly on an empty stomach. If you have kidney or liver problems, these medications may be discontinued or started at low doses.

If the tablet has "XL, SR or XR," which means extended release, do not break or cut the tablet.

Insulin Secretagogue class: These medications are known as *Prandin (repaglinide)* and *Starlix (nateglinide)*. This type of medication stimulates insulin to be produced from the pancreatic cells. However, it works faster and doesn't stay active as long as the other sulfonylureas mentioned above. This type of medication is taken immediately prior to the meal. If a meal is missed, then the dose should be skipped also. People with liver disease should use with caution.

Biguanides class: This medication is known as *metformin*, with common name brands such as *Glucophage* and *Fortamet*. Metformin improves glucose tolerance in people with Type 2 diabetes. Metformin decreases the liver's production of glucose and improves the body's sensitivity to insulin. This drug is now available in generic form. A side effect of metformin is that it can decrease appetite, which causes some people to lose a modest amount of weight. This medication is usually taken 1 to 2 times a day. When first starting on this medication, you may experience diarrhea and nausea. Generally, starting metformin slowly can minimize this. Most people tolerate this medication very well. Metformin should not be used in people with kidney or liver problems. Because this drug is excreted by the kidneys, if you need a procedure or X-ray that requires IV dye, you might be asked to stop metformin for several days after the test and have lab work checked. In females in whom ovulation might occur, precautions to avoid pregnancy should be considered.

Thiazolidinedione class: These medications, known as ***Actos (pioglitazone)*** and ***Avandia (rosiglitazone),*** help decrease insulin resistance by improving sensitivity to insulin in the muscle and fat tissue. They also help moderately decrease the liver's production of glucose. These medications are usually taken 1-2 times a day. You will be asked to have lab work checked periodically to monitor liver function while on this medication. Edema and weight gain can be a potential side effect of these medications. People with liver problems and heart failure might not be candidates for this type of medication. When this medication is combined with other medications for diabetes, there is an increased risk for low blood sugar.

Alpha-glucosidase inhibitor class: Known as ***Precose (acarbose)*** and ***Glyset (miglitol)*** these medications help slow down the breakdown of food with carbohydrates into glucose in the gut. This medication, which is taken just before a meal, helps control the after eating elevation in glucose. Side effects, which may include diarrhea and flatulence, are relatively common but not unbearable. Medications that require a steady absorption rate should not be taken at the same time such as digoxin, birth control, thyroid or phenytoin, to name a few. **To treat low blood sugar, oral glucose (dextrose) must be used and you should carry it at all times.** Glucose tablets are available at all pharmacies for a low cost. Other foods such as milk and juice will not be effective if taking alpha-glucosidase inhibitors.

Insulin is available for all people who have poor control of glucose levels. Insulin can be used in both Type 1 and Type 2 diabetes. Several insulin types are available, and each has its own rate and length of action. Insulin injections are relatively painless and easy to administer. Insulin needs to be taken about the same time each day, generally in relationship to food intake. All insulin should be stored in the refrigerator, but the bottle that is being used may be left at room temperature up to 28 days and then thrown away. Insulin comes in vials and preloaded pen devices. Insulin is safe to use in insulin pumps. Some of the insulin products that are available include Humalog, Novolog, Apidra, Regular, NPH, Lantus, and Levemir.

Although all insulin used to be taken via injection, there is a new, inhalable form of insulin called *Exubera*. After inhalation of Exubera, the meal should be eaten immediately, as the peak effects occur in approximately 2 hours and last about 6 hours. Exubera can be used in people with Type 1 or 2 diabetes. Exubera does not take the place of all insulin, and injected insulin may need to also be taken. The absorption of Exubera is affected by smoking and exposure to secondhand smoke. If you smoke, you cannot use Exubera. A person with lung disease, such as asthma or COPD, is not recommended to use inhaled insulin. A pulmonary function test is required before and after use of Exubera.

Incretin class has recently become available: Byetta* and *Symlin*. *Byetta (exenatide) is used for people with Type 2 diabetes to help lower the after-eating high glucose levels by enhancing the secretion of insulin in response to the food being eaten and assist in decreasing the liver's production of glucose. This medication is given by injection twice a day, before breakfast and evening meals. It comes in a pen device which helps with dosing and ease of taking. Byetta helps slow gastric emptying so you feel full longer. By overeating, the side effect most likely will be nausea and bloating. Eating half the amount of food normally eaten at a meal helps minimize this effect. Since eating smaller amounts of food is encouraged with Byetta, most people have a modest weight loss.

Symlin (pramlintide acetate) is used for people with Type 1 or 2 diabetes who are using insulin. Symlin replaces some of the actions of a hormone called amylin, which is thought to be lacking in people with diabetes who use insulin. Symlin, which helps to lower blood sugars after the meal is eaten, must be injected no more than 15 minutes prior to every meal. Like Byetta, Symlin helps with the rate the stomach empties, decreases the amount of sugar the liver produces, and helps decrease appetite. Symlin can produce low blood sugars, therefore, the current insulin dose is reduced initially when Symlin is started. Close monitoring of blood sugars is required when starting this medication. Symlin and insulin should not be mixed together in the same syringe. Symlin can produce nausea and vomiting as a possible side effect. Weight loss is also possible with Symlin. People with **gastroparesis** (slow motility of their stomach) or stomach disorders should not take either Byetta or Symlin.

Januvia (sitagliptin) was approved by the FDA in 2006 for the treatment of diabetes. Januvia helps to increase the active levels of Incretin hormones by inhibiting an enzyme called DPP4. Incretin hormones are released by the intestine, which helps to regulate glucose stabilization. Januvia is used only for patients with Type 2 diabetes and is given orally once a day. This medication may also be combined with other oral diabetes medications. People with kidney disease may need lower doses of this medication. Januvia does not enhance weight loss.

Should I exercise if I have diabetes?

Yes, you should exercise daily! Exercise can help control diabetes by increasing muscle mass, which can help with insulin resistance and weight control. The American Diabetes Association recommends 30-45 minutes of moderate aerobic activity daily, with a goal of at least 150 minutes total per week. If there are physical limitations, these can be overcome by looking at a variety of activities such as a stationary bike, treadmill, swimming, water aerobics, walking or arm-chair exercises. If you have other health challenges, then you may need to discuss plans to participate in a physical exercise program with your health care provider. Remember, exercise generally helps most diseases. Many fitness centers offer exercises for the older adult that provide not only a good, safe exercise program but a chance to make friends.

Before exercising, check your blood sugar to make sure it is normal, at or above 100. Always carry something to treat low blood sugar with you at all times because exercise can bring on hypoglycemia or low blood sugar (blood sugar below 70). If you experience low blood sugar on exercise days, your medication may need to be adjusted before participating or a small snack may be needed.

What is hypoglycemia, or low blood sugar?

Anyone taking diabetes medication can have *hypoglycemia*, or *low blood sugar*. Hypoglycemia is a blood sugar that is lower than 70.

Symptoms may include:
- Sweating
- Hunger
- Unclear thinking
- Lightheadedness
- Unsteadiness
- Trembling
- Weakness
- Nervousness

Causes of low blood sugar are usually related to one of three things: food, activity or medication. For example, if you are doing extra housework or yard work, you may be at an increased risk for developing low blood sugar due to increased activity. Skipping breakfast to eat a big lunch with friends would put you at an increased risk for low blood sugar in the morning before lunch. This is an example of food-related low blood sugar. Most people will have low blood sugar occasionally if they are on diabetes medications. However, low blood sugar should be quickly treated and should never be allowed to get to the point of losing consciousness. Low blood sugar generally has symptoms that occur rapidly; however with aging it can be harder to feel low blood sugar. Therefore, it is important to check your blood sugar if you are having symptoms, in order to verify if your sugar is below 70 or not. If you are having these symptoms and your sugar level is above 70, there may be something else causing it and you need to see your health care provider. The only way you know if you are having a low blood sugar is to verify it with a home blood glucose test.

Treatment: If your sugar level is under 70, then you need to eat or drink 15 to 20 grams of carbohydrate. Chose **one** of the following to treat low blood sugar below 70:

- 3-4 Glucose tablets
- 4-6 oz. of fruit juice
- 10 Lifesavers (chew and swallow)
- 4-6 oz. of regular soda (NOT diet)
- 8 oz. of milk

After treating a low blood sugar, wait 15-20 minutes, then recheck your blood sugar reading to make sure your blood sugar has returned to normal, generally above 100.

Anyone taking diabetes medications should at *all times carry sugar* such as glucose tablets or hard candy.

Using other food items such as bread or candy bars is not recommended to treat low blood sugar since they take longer to digest and have extra calories not needed.

Older adults are at a higher risk for low blood sugar due to kidney changes, irregular food intake, multiple medications, inadequate fluid intake, and changes in intestinal absorption. You need to ask your health care provider what is the lowest you should keep your glucose readings. You may be asked to keep your blood sugars slightly higher to help avoid the risk of having low blood sugar. **If you have low blood sugar during the night, get up and treat it immediately. Do not try to go back to sleep without treating it.** Always retest your blood sugar one hour after treating it in the middle of the night. Keep glucose at your bedside at all times that you can reach easily. Glucose tablets and hard candy work well to keep at the bedside since they don't require refrigeration.

I never eat sweets, so why are my blood sugars high, and why can't I lose weight?

Food issues are probably one of the most frequently asked questions since food is used every day and there are so many choices. Many people need to make better food choices; be it amount or the type of food eaten to have a healthier lifestyle. While genetics can play a role in obesity, you are still responsible for what and how much you eat. There are no "miracles" to losing weight, other than increase physical activity (burning up energy) and decrease the amount of calories eaten (energy intake). The human body needs a variety of food sources – meat, fruit, starch and vegetables – to be healthy. Any diet that leaves out an entire food group is probably a bad idea. So take this into consideration when attempting to change your dietary intake.

Carbohydrates are the main contributor of glucose to your diet. Because they are an excellent food source for energy, carbohydrates should not be avoided totally. While limiting sweets and desserts is a good habit, do not forget other sources of carbohydrates such as bread, pasta (noodles/rice), milk, fruit and grains. Most of us eat too many carbohydrates, and this affects the blood sugar directly. That is why you have been asked to limit your portions of pasta, fruit, juice and milk on a daily basis.

While it is vitally important to watch the carbohydrate intake, it is also important not to forget the other nutrients. Protein is needed for muscle and tissue growth, and is a possible energy supply. Some of our protein comes from meat, dairy, beans, nuts, seeds and legumes. Eating protein has minimal effects on blood sugars.

A variety of vegetables is needed to obtain the vitamins and minerals needed. Most vegetables are excellent sources of fiber and are relatively low in calories. The majority of vegetables do not contribute to blood sugars. Vegetables generally can be eaten relatively freely except for a few starchy vegetables, such as peas, potatoes and corn. Starchy vegetables are healthy, but need to be measured and counted as carbohydrates.

Fats are also a needed food nutrient, but in very small amounts. Unfortunately, the typical American diet has too much fat. Too much fat contributes to the development of Type 2 diabetes, heart disease and obesity. Many of our protein sources naturally have fat in them, such as meat, nuts, seeds, dairy and eggs; therefore, there is little need to add extra fat to the diet. Fat and protein do not contribute directly to the blood glucose level; however, since they do contribute calories, they should be eaten in moderation. Fat has more than two times as many calories per gram when compared to protein and carbohydrates.

The key to any diet/lifestyle change is an awareness of what and how much is actually eaten on any given day. A successful weight loss tool that is affordable for every one is the food record or diary (the cost is a piece of paper and a pen.) A food diary can help you identify all of the carbohydrates that are eaten, which inadvertently raise your glucose level. It can also help you identify areas where too much or the wrong foods are eaten, as well. So get out your measuring cups/spoons and **measure everything** that goes into your mouth for at least 4 days! It will require measuring your cereal, milk, corn, mashed potatoes, etc. Don't forget to include snacks, even if it is 1 or 2 pretzels. Write down everything you eat or drink, including sugar-free items, in your diary.

Example of a Food Diary:

Breakfast	Oatmeal packet *
	¾ cup milk *
	1 cup juice *
	Coffee-cream
Snack	3 graham crackers *
	Sugar-free cocoa*
Lunch	Tuna salad sandwich*
	Chips-21 *
	Diet soda
	Apple-medium *

Then, "look up" the foods to see what has carbohydrates. Don't forget to look up the calories and portion sizes too! There are many resources available to look up carbohydrates and other nutrient values that are free on the Internet or at your local library. Note in the example, the * sign beside the foods indicates that food item had carbohydrates. Read the food labels on the boxes and cans; all have portion sizes, and the amount of carbohydrates, but don't get so focused on carbohydrates that calories are forgotten. Calorie intake should not be ignored for most adults. Remember: too many calories, regardless of what the food is, will make you too fat!

Learning about food can be complicated, so if you are still having trouble with managing your diabetes, ask your health

care provider to recommend a **registered dietitian.**
Good luck!

How often do I need an eye exam since I have diabetes?

Every person should have a ***dilated eye*** exam soon after being diagnosed with diabetes. After the initial exam, generally a yearly dilated exam is recommended. If eye problems are seen at the exam, then you may be asked to be seen more frequently. ***Glaucoma***, ***cataracts*** and ***retinopathy*** are more common in people with diabetes, so it is important to have regular eye exams. You cannot see or feel these changes, so regular exams are recommended. ***Diabetic retinopathy*** involves blood vessel changes in the back of the eye that only your optometrist or ophthalmologist can see. Diabetic retinopathy is thought to be one of the most common causes of blindness and must be taken seriously. Treatment is available to help decrease the damage of retinopathy, but prevention by having good diabetes control is the best way.

How do I know if I have kidney damage (nephropathy) from my diabetes?

Diabetes can cause damage to the kidneys (***nephropathy***) that cannot be felt. A simple urine test called a ***microalbuminuria test*** should be done yearly, which can be done right in your health care provider's office. A blood test called a ***serum creatinine*** can also be done annually to test for the ***glomerular filtration rate (GFR)***. The GFR test can be used to help determine how well your kidneys are working.

Unfortunately, it is estimated 20-40% of people with diabetes have kidney damage. Having good blood sugar and blood pressure control can help decrease the rate of kidney damage. There are two types of blood pressure medications that have been shown to help reduce the risk of kidney damage and of heart disease as well. These types of blood pressure medications are called *ACE inhibitors* or *ARB's*. If you can not tolerate one, the other one is generally well-tolerated. Controlling blood pressure is vitally important to helping maintain kidney function. To reduce the risk of kidney and heart damage, many people may need to take several blood pressure medications at the same time. It is vitally important to take your blood pressure medication daily to protect your kidneys.

My feet hurt . . . could it be from diabetes?

Diabetes can cause a condition called *neuropathy*. Neuropathy is nerve damage which most commonly is caused from diabetes. Symptoms of neuropathy can range from barely noticeable to severe pain. Generally people will complain about their feet feeling cold, numb or tingling off and on. On rare occasions, the symptoms of neuropathy can progress to feeling like electrical shocks, shooting or burning pain. Neuropathy pain generally starts in the toes and feet and occasionally will go to the hands. Neuropathy can affect all organs. This condition can get worse over time, and there is no good treatment to prevent neuropathy except having good control of your blood sugars. There are medications that can be used to help control neuropathy pain. A person with neuropathy in the feet needs to be very careful to protect the feet. Wear protective shoes, which are proper fitting (do not pinch the toes or bunions). If you notice red areas or callouses, most likely it is caused from your shoe rubbing, an indication that the shoe does not fit correctly. In this case, you are advised to throw the shoes away and get new ones! Having diabetic neuropathy puts you at a high risk for development of foot ulcers, which can lead to amputation. A cute or expensive pair of shoes is not worth losing your foot! Every time you see health care providers, take your shoes and socks off so your feet can be examined. Your feet should be screened annually for diabetic neuropathy by your healthcare provider. If you ever notice a sore or open area on your foot, immediately seek medical help.

What if I have the flu and diabetes?

It is important to maintain hydration during an illness. It is important to drink at least 4 to 8 ounces of calorie-free liquids every hour. Examples of calorie-free drinks include diet soft drink, water and broth. Liquids with sodium and electrolytes should be consumed every 3 hours. Bouillon, canned clear broth, Gatorade, and Pedialyte are some examples of fluids with electrolytes. If you have a fluid or sodium restriction due to heart or kidney problems, please check with your health care provider on the amount you should take. Blood sugars frequently are elevated with illness; therefore, monitor your blood sugars every 2-4 hours during illness. It is important to write down your blood sugars during this time, because if you need medical assistance, you may be asked about your blood sugar readings. If you are vomiting and not tolerating fluids with high blood sugars, you may be asked to complete a urine test for ketones at home. If vomiting cannot be controlled, you may need to go to the emergency room.

Insulin and/or most diabetes pills are still needed even if you are ill. If you take insulin, skipping insulin totally may cause a condition called *ketosis (a condition where high acid content is found in the blood)*. In general, insulin will be required during your illness. On occasion, if an illness persists, insulin may be needed by people who normally take oral medication for diabetes. If a person is taking metformin and is seriously ill, metformin may be stopped temporarily.

Due to nausea, soft foods are frequently tolerated better during an illness. Attempting to take 45-50 grams of carbohydrate every 2-3 hours is a general guideline.

Examples of 15 grams of carbohydrate:
½ cup clear juice, such as apple
½ cup regular soda
1 slice toast
6 saltine crackers
1 cup sports drink (e.g., Gatorade)
½ cup regular gelatin
½ cup Cream of Wheat
3 squares graham crackers
1 full Popsicle bar

When do I call my health care provider or go to the emergency room?

- Vomiting lasting longer than 6 hours, or vomiting more than 3-4 times in a row without keeping anything down in-between
- Moderate to large ketones
- Blood sugar level over 300 on 2 consecutive measurements, 1 hour or more apart
- After you have received *glucagon* injection

If you are ill, do not hesitate to call your health care provider for instructions.

I have been told to go to diabetes education . . . do I have to go?

Yes, since diabetes is a chronic condition that will be with you for the rest of your life, it is important to take the time to learn how to manage it. Look for a Certified Diabetes Educator (CDE) to be assured of quality diabetes education. CDE's offer classes to individuals and groups for the purpose of learning to take care of yourself and managing your disease. Your family is welcome and encouraged to attend education sessions with you. While your spouse, "significant other" or other family member may do the cooking, you are responsible for what and how much you eat, so you need to see the dietitian too. Medicare and many insurance companies now help pay for diabetes education, since it is so important. Remember, you are in control of your diet, activity and medication, so it is up to you to learn how to manage diabetes.

"It's up to you . . ."
Diabetes is a relentless disease that never gives a break or holiday. Unfortunately, it must be managed 24 hours a day, but fortunately we have many wonderful treatments and ways to help you manage it and make your life easier. If you have a healthy lifestyle that uses diet and exercise as the backbone to diabetes management, and take your medications, you will greatly increase your chances to have a better quality of life.

Osteoporosis: a Leading Cause of Bone Fracture as We Grow Older
Susan Freburg, ARNP

A 65-year old woman breaks her wrist after slipping on ice. Should she ask for a bone density test and an evaluation for osteoporosis even if her health care provider doesn't bring it up?

Yes! Strong bones are essential to good health and allow older adults the ability to enjoy life at its fullest. Yet, too many adults suffer from *fractures (broken bones)* that often lead to a decline in physical and mental well being. Fractures not only cause pain and disability but also contribute to loss of independence and even death. Many of these fractures could be prevented. Understanding the importance of good nutrition, physical activity and healthy lifestyle choices will help you take steps to improve bone health and reduce your risk of fractures.

What is bone health?
The *bony skeleton* provides a frame for the body that allows for movement and protects vital organs. In addition, it stores

and *phosphorus*. To respond to its dual roles of support and regulation of calcium and phosphorus, and to repair any damage to the skeleton, bone is constantly undergoing change by a process known as *remodeling*. Remodeling allows both active bone formation and breakdown throughout life so that most of the adult skeleton is replaced about every 10 years. Remodeling repairs any damage the skeleton incurs by replacing small cracks with new bone, which restores bone strength. Healthy bone is maintained when the amount of bone formation is equal to the rate of bone breakdown. In aging adults and individuals with other risks, the rate of bone breakdown exceeds the rate of bone formation and can result in significant loss of bone mass.

What is osteoporosis?

Osteoporosis is "a skeletal disorder characterized by compromised bone strength, predisposing to an increased risk of fracture" (NIH Consensus Statement 2000). The word osteoporosis literally means *bone (osteo) that is filled with holes (porosis)*. Osteoporosis is the most common bone disease and is the major cause of bone fractures in women following menopause and in older adults.

There are two types of osteoporosis, primary and secondary.

Primary osteoporosis is responsible for approximately 80% of cases and is thought to be related to estrogen deficiency in women (known as postmenopausal osteoporosis) and the aging process. In primary osteoporosis, bone is broken down faster than it is replaced. This leads to progressive erosion of bone and bone loss. Bones with less mass are more likely to break, even with a minor fall.

Secondary osteoporosis is associated with a specific, underlying cause and leads to greater amounts of bone loss than a normal individual would experience. Several medical conditions and prescription medications can affect bone health. Some medical conditions related to secondary osteoporosis include hyperthyroidism, chronic lung disease, cancer, inflammatory bowel disease, chronic liver or kidney disease, rheumatoid arthritis, hyperparathyroidism and vitamin D deficiency. Some medications known to contribute to the development of osteoporosis include oral glucocorticoids (steroids), cancer treatments, thyroid medication, antiepileptic medication, gonadal hormones and immunosuppresive agents. Secondary causes of the disease are common in women who have not reached menopause and in the majority of men with osteoporosis. In addition, it is estimated that up to a third of postmenopausal women with osteoporosis also have other conditions that may contribute to their bone loss.

How common is osteoporosis?

The Surgeon General's report on bone health (October 2004), found that **10 million Americans over the age of 50 have osteoporosis**. Approximately 1.5 million fractures (broken bones) related to osteoporosis occur every year.

Other findings in the report include:
- About 20 percent of senior citizens who suffer a hip fracture die within a year of fracture.
- About 20 percent of individuals with a hip fracture end up in a nursing home within a year.
- Hip fractures account for 300,000 hospitalizations each year.

Estimates project that by 2020, half of all American citizens older than 50 will be at risk for fractures from osteoporosis and low bone mass if individuals at risk are not identified and treated. These predictions are not likely to decrease unless preventive actions are taken.

Am I at risk for osteoporosis?

A dangerous myth about osteoporosis is that it only affects women. **Osteoporosis affects both men and women of all races.** Approximately one-fourth of all hip fractures occur in men. Too many assume they are not at risk for bone loss or fractures.

Check any of these that apply to you:

- ☐ I'm older than 65.
- ☐ I've broken a bone after age 50.
- ☐ My close relative has osteoporosis or has broken a bone.
- ☐ My health is "fair" or "poor."
- ☐ I smoke.
- ☐ I am underweight for my height.
- ☐ I started menopause before age 45.
- ☐ I've had low calcium intake.
- ☐ I have more than two alcohol drinks several times a week.
- ☐ I have poor vision, even with glasses.
- ☐ I sometimes fall.
- ☐ I'm not active.
- ☐ I have a medical condition or take a medication associated with bone loss (listed in above section *What is osteoporosis?*)

If one or more of these factors apply to you, you are at greater risk for developing osteoporosis and breaking a bone.

What are the symptoms of osteoporosis?

Osteoporosis is often described as a "silent thief" because the loss of bone mass occurs without symptoms. Many people already have weak bones and don't know it. Fragile bones are not painful at first. The first warning sign of osteoporosis may be a broken bone.

A broken bone that results from a low-trauma fall is considered a *fragility (osteoporotic) fracture*. A *low-trauma fracture* is defined by the World Health Organization as a broken bone that results from a fall from standing height or less. The types of broken bones most often involved are the wrist, hip, upper arm or shoulder and back.

The most common osteoporotic fracture is a spine fracture, which is 2 to 3 times more common than hip fractures. Only 33% experience pain, and the remainder of spine fractures are often undetected. Spine fractures can result in a loss of height, postural changes, rounded shoulders, and reduced quality of life. Up to half of those with a spine fracture will experience additional spine fractures within 3 years, many within the first year. A prior spine fracture increases the risk of other types of fractures by 2 to 3 times.

Most hip fractures are caused by falling from a standing height; only about 5% occur *before* a person falls. Following a hip fracture, a person over the age of 65 has a 20% likelihood of dying in one year. Among those who survived, another 20% will lose their independency and are placed in long-term care homes. Nearly 65,000 American women die of complications from hip fractures each year.

Fractures of the wrist or forearm typically occur outdoors in winter and are caused by falling on an outstretched hand. The mortality (death) rate is low, but other complications such as pain, temporary disability and degenerative arthritis are high.

Fractures from osteoporosis can happen in almost any bone in the body. Once a fragility fracture has occurred, the chance for more fractures greatly increases.

Do you know your T-Score?

Many believe that if we haven't had any signs of bone damage, then our bones are strong. Most of us have our blood pressure and cholesterol checked for heart health. One of the best ways to know if you have osteoporosis is through

bone mineral density testing (DXA).   Bone mineral testing helps identify individuals at risk prior to a bone fracture.

Bone density testing is painless, quick (5 to 10 minutes) and safe.   The results of your bone mineral test are compared to the average bone density recorded for healthy, young adult women as a ***T-Score***.

Here is what your T-score means:
>**Above -1**: Your bone density is considered normal.
>**Between -1 and -2.5**: Your score is a sign of low bone mass, this means your bone density is below normal and may lead to osteoporosis.
>**Below -2.5**: Your bone density indicates you have osteoporosis.

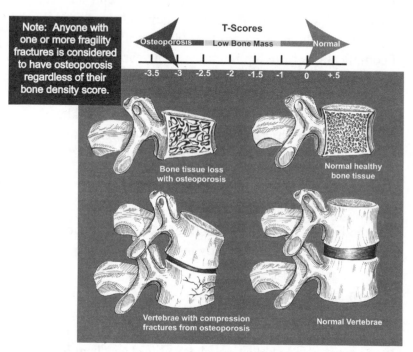

Figure 1. Normal vertebrae vs. vertebrae with osteoporosis with T-Score values (*T-score scale is based on a similar scale provided by ORA, Davenport, Iowa*)

What is low bone mass, or osteopenia?

Low bone mass and *osteopenia* are terms describing the results of a bone mineral testing measurement (DXA). Low bone mass (osteopenia) is not a disease, but it can lead to the development of osteoporosis and place an individual at increased risk of fracture, particularly if other risk factors are present.

What are the causes of bone loss and fractures in osteoporosis?

Many things can interfere with the development of a strong and healthy skeleton. *Genetics* and *lifestyle choices* contribute to bone loss and the development of osteoporosis.

Bone mass increases throughout the first three decades of life, reaching its peak around age 30. Peak bone mass is primarily determined by genetics but may be influenced by other factors such as *physical activity, diet (inadequate calcium intake), medical conditions* and *lifestyle choices (tobacco and alcohol use)*. Osteoporosis is more likely to develop if peak bone mass is not achieved at skeletal maturity.

After achieving peak bone mass, bone formation remains equal to bone breakdown until about age 40, when bone mass begins to decline slowly.

Once menopause begins, women begin to lose bone mass rapidly, and for approximately 5 to 7 years may lose as much as a third of their bone mass (Arthritis Foundation). Women are also at greater risk of losing bone mass than men because they have about 30 percent less bone mass than men at the time of peak bone mass.

After the age of 70, both men and women experience *accelerated bone loss* and the *inability to build new bone*.

Other factors influence bone mass. ***Lack of physical activity*** tends to decrease bone mass. A ***diet low in calcium, phosphorus and vitamin D*** is associated with bone loss. The ***use of caffeine, alcohol and tobacco*** all can contribute to decreased bone mass. ***Menstrual cycles that begin late*** in girls and ***early menopause*** also place women at increased risk for bone loss and the development of osteoporosis.

While low bone mass may put an individual at risk of fracture, it is often the fall that accounts for the injury. **Falls are one of the most common problems that threaten the independence of older individuals.** An increased tendency to fall occurs with aging due to ***loss of muscle strength***, ***poor vision*** or ***medications that impair balance***. *Remember, it isn't the fall that hurts, it's the sudden stop*!

What can I do to keep my bones healthy?

The good news is that you are never too old or too young to improve your bone health. **The keys to preventing osteoporosis are building strong bone and preventing bone loss.** While you have no control over genetics, you can prevent or slow down osteoporosis by making wise lifestyle choices.

Increase your calcium intake to at least 1200 mg daily either through diet or calcium supplements. When calcium intake isn't adequate, the body draws calcium from the bones to keep blood levels normal. ***Dairy products*** provide the best source of calcium-rich foods. If enough calcium is not obtained through the diet, ***calcium supplements*** should be used to achieve the recommended daily requirements. A single dose should not exceed 600 mg of elemental calcium. Calcium supplements are available in a variety of salts with different concentrations of elemental calcium. ***Calcium citrate*** can be taken with or without food.

Calcium carbonate should be taken with food to improve absorption.

Obtain the recommended minimum daily requirement of vitamin D of 400-800 IU/daily. *Vitamin D* increases the amount of calcium your body absorbs. Your body produces vitamin D in response to exposure to *sunlight*. It is not widely available in natural food sources. It is primarily found in *fish oils*, some *vegetables*, and *fortified milk, cereals and breads*. Older adults are at increased risk for *vitamin D deficiency* because they often do not receive adequate sun exposure and vitamin D absorption may be reduced.

Remain physically active with regular weight-bearing and muscle-strengthening exercise. An exercise program that increases the force of gravity on your bones can strengthen and maintain bone mass. Many activities are enjoyable and promote bone health, such as aerobics, dancing, tennis and walking. Regular exercise also improves balance and mobility, which may help prevent falls.

Avoid smoking and excess alcohol. People who smoke have a 55% increase in hip fracture risk. Smoking reduces bone mass in several ways. Smokers tend to weigh less, experience menopause earlier and have reduced calcium absorption. Those who drink more than two alcoholic drinks a day have a higher risk of developing osteoporosis because they have less bone mass and lose bone more rapidly. The risk of bone fractures is higher because alcohol use increases the chance of falling.

Prevent falls by having regular vision checks, avoid medications that may cause dizziness or confusion, and make sure your home is safe. Suggestions for making your home safer and reducing your chance for falling include *eliminating throw rugs and clutter, making sure hallways,*

109

stairwells and entrances are well lit, installing handrails in bathrooms, halls and stairways, and **wearing sturdy, low-heeled shoes with non-slip soles**. For those at highest risk for falling and breaking a bone, additional precautions might include physical therapy or the use of hip protectors.

What medications can treat osteoporosis and help prevent bone fractures?

Very effective medications are available and can significantly reduce the risk of a broken bone. There are two primary types of medication.

Antiresorptive therapies include the **bisphosphonates**, **estrogen**, **selective estrogen receptor modulators (SERM)** and **calcitonin**. These therapies decrease the risk of fractures by reducing bone loss, decreasing bone turnover and stabilizing bone structure. Three **Food and Drug Administration (FDA)**-approved bisphosphonates are available: **alendronate**, **risedronate** and **ibandronate**. Only one SERM, **raloxifene**, is FDA-approved. Although **estrogen therapy** is effective for the prevention of postmenopausal osteoporosis, it should only be considered for women at significant risk of osteoporosis who cannot take non-estrogen medications. The decision to use hormone therapy must take into consideration the increased risk of other health problems, **including increased risk of stroke**, **cognitive impairment**, **blood clots** and **breast cancer**. **Calcitonin** is less effective than other antiresorptive therapies but is well-tolerated and provides pain relief in spine fractures.

Anabolic therapy is available for individuals who are at high risk for fractures or lose bone while on antiresorptive therapy. **Teriparatide (PTH)** is a synthetic form of **parathyroid hormone** and is the only FDA-approved anabolic agent. Unlike other available agents, **Teriparitide** works by stimulating new bone formation. **Teriparitide** is given by subcutaneous injection over two years and increases bone strength by thickening the outer shell of bones and increasing the connections within the bony structures of the skeleton.

Conclusion

Thirty years ago, little was known about bone disease. Bone mineral density testing (DXA) was not available and effective treatments had not been discovered. Many people believed that weak and broken bones were a natural part of growing old. This is no longer true! Much is known about how to keep bone healthy throughout life and how to prevent and treat bone disease and bone fractures. In the past 15 years, research has identified important risk factors in developing osteoporosis. Bone mineral density testing (DXA) is available to identify people at risk *before* a broken bone occurs.

If you have osteoporosis, several additional steps should be taken. A comprehensive evaluation by your health care professional should be performed and include special blood tests to determine whether you have treatable factors contributing to your osteoporosis. Effective medications are available that prevent bone breakdown (antiresorptives) or build new bone (anabolics). Medication treatment should be considered in everyone who has osteoporosis especially when a broken bone has occurred.

You can live life to the fullest and prevent the devastating consequences of bone fractures and osteoporosis by paying attention to the basics – eating a healthy diet, exercising regularly, avoiding the use of tobacco and alcohol and taking action to prevent falls.

Cholesterol, Aging and Heart Disease
Peter P. Toth, MD, PhD, FAAFP, FCCP, FAHA, FACC

The *population* of the United States is aging. This demographic change is attributable to the fact that both men and women and people of all racial and ethnic groups are living longer. The *average life expectancy* has increased nearly two-fold since the time of our great-grandparents. During the first half of the 20th Century, much of this increase in *longevity* was due to improved sanitation, the development of vaccines and antibiotics and improved working conditions. Since approximately 1960, *life expectancies* have continued to increase secondary to the development of radically new life-saving drugs and technologies in cardiovascular medicine. Far and away, modern cardiology has raised expectations about the quality and quantity of life people can expect to experience. Each of us strives to get the most out of life. One very important issue pertaining to longevity and health is to know your cholesterol level and to get help if it is abnormal.

What is cholesterol?
Cholesterol is a fat-like substance found in our blood and cells. There are three forms of cholesterol, forms that can be conveniently labeled as "the good, the bad and the ugly."

The *"good" cholesterol* is *HDL*, or *"high-density lipoprotein cholesterol."* The *"bad" cholesterol* is *LDL*, or *"low-density lipoprotein."* The *"ugly" cholesterol* is *Lp(a)*, or *lipoprotein(a)*.

How is cholesterol measured, and what do cholesterol readings indicate?
The amount of cholesterol in your blood is determined by

your genetic constitution and your diet. Until recently, it was believed that a total cholesterol level less than 200 mg/dL was *a "normal" cholesterol reading*. However, we now know that it is much more important to look at different components of your cholesterol profile, namely the *LDL (bad cholesterol)*, *HDL (good cholesterol)*, and *triglycerides (blood fats)*.

In order to increase the odds that you will live longer and without heart disease, it is advisable that you keep your bad cholesterol low and your good cholesterol high. An optimal LDL is less than 100 mg/dL. However, if you have had a heart attack or are a diabetic with coronary disease, you should try to get your LDL below 70 mg/dL.

Dropping your LDL to very low levels generally requires medication and lifestyle modification, including exercise and significant dietary changes. A man should try to keep his HDL above 40 mg/dL, while a woman should keep her HDL above 50 mg/dL. Mounting evidence from studies conducted in Europe and the United States suggests that in people older than 70 years, HDL becomes an even more important risk factor than your LDL. Your health care provider should not ignore your HDL or downplay its significance. As a rule, triglycerides should be kept below 150 mg/dL.

All risk factors increase in prevalence as populations age. Cholesterol, blood pressure, diabetes, and obesity all tend to increase with age. As we get older, our risk for heart attack, stroke, sudden death (dropping dead from a heart attack), carotid artery and peripheral artery disease and heart failure all increase significantly. Much of this is due to long-term wear and tear. As we age, our blood vessels are exposed to the profound stress imposed by elevated cholesterol, blood pressure, high blood sugar levels, and, sometimes, cigarette smoke, to name a few of the most important risk

114

factors. Decreasing bad cholesterol and triglyceride levels, blood pressure, blood sugar if you are diabetic, and smoking cessation are all protective to your blood vessels and decrease the rate at which your cardiovascular system ages and develops disease.

What is atherosclerosis?

The process of *atherosclerosis (hardening of the arteries)* begins in childhood and adolescence. Unfortunate young men who were killed in combat during the conflicts in Korea and Vietnam already often showed evidence of significant coronary artery disease by the time they were in their late teens and early 20's. Developing coronary disease is no longer inevitable. However, most people older than 45 or 50 harbor some degree of disease if one looks closely enough. Consequently, as a rule of thumb, the sooner your particular collection of risk factors for heart disease is identified, the sooner they can be treated so that your risk for cardiovascular disease can be decreased. We are learning that if risk factors such as cholesterol are treated very aggressively, we can actually begin to see tangible evidence that blood vessel walls begin to heal and disease reverses. Accompanying these changes, we find that risk for heart attack, stroke and death all decrease significantly.

What exactly does cholesterol do to your heart and blood vessels?

Good question! The answer is, as we have come to expect in medicine, quite complicated. We have labeled LDL the "bad cholesterol" because it induces the net deposit of cholesterol in blood vessels throughout the body. LDL is actually a transport vehicle of sorts for cholesterol. But it is a dump truck. You really do not want cholesterol dumped into your blood vessels because the progressive dumping of this substance leads to the progressive narrowing of blood

115

vessels, eventually choking off blood flow to critical organs such as your heart muscle, brain, kidney, or legs.

HDL is the good cholesterol because it is the great biological custodian: it mops up after your LDL. It promotes the mobilization of cholesterol from your blood vessels and transports cholesterol back to the liver for elimination through your intestines. The more HDL you have, the lower your odds of developing heart disease. Raising your good cholesterol and dropping your bad cholesterol are the primary goals your doctor has in managing your cholesterol balance. Similar to LDL, triglycerides also tend to plug your blood vessels. True to form, your HDL can help to clean these troublemakers up as well.

How do diet and exercise influence cholesterol levels?

Dietary interventions *(diet)* can beneficially impact your cholesterol levels. Decreasing your consumption of saturated fat (generally animal fat) and trans fat will decrease your LDL.

Exercise has been shown to decrease LDL, raise HDL and relieve insulin resistance and thereby lower your blood sugar.

The Mediterranean diet emphasizes the consumption of whole grains, legumes, fruits, vegetables, and olive oil, and is associated with beneficial changes in all of your cholesterol panel components. This diet is also associated with weight loss and reduced risk for developing diabetes.

What else can we do to positively affect our cholesterol?

Weight loss, *smoking cessation* and the *consumption of walnut or flaxseed oil* are associated with increased blood levels of HDL.

Which medications are available to optimize cholesterol levels?

If your cholesterol numbers are out of sorts, there are numerous medications we can use to help you optimize them. The most important drugs for treating cholesterol are the *statins* (i.e., *Crestor, Lipitor, Zocor, Lescol, Pravachol, Mevacor*). The statins decrease cholesterol by inhibiting cholesterol production by the liver. Although these drugs tend to be maligned by the press and on the Internet, they save lives. The statins have been used to treat millions of people around the world and their ability to decrease heart attack, stroke, death and even the frequency of anginal chest pain is intensively studied and documented. Contrary to what you hear, these drugs have never been shown to cause liver failure. More recent data shows that they can even improve kidney function. They can cause *muscle aching* (*myalgia*), but generally this can be treated by dropping the dose for a while or switching to a different statin.

Your doctor will check your liver tests (via a blood sample) twice per year to ensure that the levels of two *liver enzymes* (*ALT* and *AST*) have not risen to a level that is greater than three times the upper limit of normal. This is an unusual development, but if it occurs, your statin will be stopped. It is unknown why this can occur in approximately 1% of patients, but often it is attributable to underlying liver disease or drug interactions. Almost as a rule, if the elevation in these tests is due to the statin, they will normalize over the next 1-3 months. A different statin should then be initiated. It is now well-accepted that if you have coronary artery disease, you have had a heart attack or stroke, or if you are diabetic, you should be on a statin. If placed on a statin, you should work carefully with your doctor to stay on it.

Other drugs to treat cholesterol are also available. ***Zetia (ezetimibe)*** is another drug that can significantly lower your bad cholesterol. It works by reducing your ability to absorb cholesterol from dietary sources. Zetia therapy allows for cholesterol to simply pass through your gastrointestinal tract. The ***fibrates (Tricor, Lopid)*** help to reduce triglycerides and raise the good cholesterol. Prescription ***niacin*** is currently the best drug available for raising HDL, but it also reduces LDL and triglycerides to a significant degree. Your doctor will tailor therapies to address the abnormalities of your ***lipid profile***. Some patients will require two or more medications to normalize their cholesterol panel.

Do we need to be careful about mixing medications and supplements?

Yes! If your good cholesterol is low, do not take vitamin E or vitamin C supplements because they can lower your good cholesterol further and impair the capacity of cholesterol drugs to raise your HDL.

Want to go natural and not take a statin? Think red rice yeast extract is the way to go? Red rice yeast extract has the capacity to lower cholesterol because it contains lovastatin, the same statin in Mevacor and one that is produced naturally by a fungus. Red rice yeast extract will not, in general, lower your cholesterol enough to make a therapeutic difference. If you need a statin, then take a statin in accordance with your doctor's recommendations.

How about fish oil enriched with omega-3 fatty acids?

Good stuff. Anyone with coronary disease should take a ***fish oil supplement*** daily (1000 mg of fish oil one to three times daily). Fish oil supplementation decreases risk for heart attack and *disturbances in your heart rhythm* (*arrhythmias*).

How frequently should cholesterol level be checked?

Your cholesterol level should be checked twice every year to insure that you are consistently meeting your therapeutic goals. The longer you stay on medication, the greater the long-term benefit. We are often asked after the first six-week follow-up visit, "Well, Doc, now that my cholesterol is good, how long do I have to stay on medication?" Answer: until something better comes out. If you stop your medication and *lifestyle modifications*, your cholesterol will go back to the way it was within just few weeks and you will lose the protection afforded to you by the medication used.

How old should you be when you start taking medication for a bad cholesterol profile?

The sooner the better and, more specifically, the younger the better, especially if you still plan on living life to the fullest and without disability when you are 80, 90, or 100 years old. Stick with the program developed in consultation with your doctor. In all likelihood, you will be glad you did. In addition to keeping you out of the emergency room because of chest pain at two o'clock in the morning, drugs that control your cholesterol have been shown to significantly drop your risk for having to undergo angioplasty and bypass surgery.

Want to live longer and with less long-term disability?

Have your doctor evaluate your *cardiovascular risk factors* in a comprehensive fashion. Get your *cholesterol, blood pressure*, and *blood sugar* screened. Allow yourself to be treated if any of these parameters is abnormal. Stop smoking, exercise, and eat healthy. Surprises can still happen. No one can issue written guarantees for living to a certain age. These relatively simple but important measures will, however, greatly increase your odds.

Chapter 10

Quitting Smoking: It is Never Too Late
Chris Pekios, RRT

Quitting smoking is hard. Why should I quit this late in life?

Quitting smoking at any time in life is a good thing. And quitting later in life has its benefits, too. The risks for, and effects on, heart disease will be reduced. That "smoker's cough" will go away, and you will have more wind to play with grandchildren. The risk for cancer takes 5-10 years to diminish, but who knows how long we will live for sure? Besides, smoking can diminish cancer-fighting treatments. Not buying tobacco products will improve your cash flow. Your house, clothes, car, and even you will smell better, too.

What are the harmful effects of tobacco use?

Cancer risks: Not just lung cancer, but larynx, esophagus, stomach, colon, and even reproductive system cancers are more common in smokers. Quitting improves the body's response to cancer-fighting treatments.

Heart disease: Smoking has been a known cause of heart disease since the 1950's. It constricts the blood vessels, increasing the blood pressure, and causes the heart to work harder and faster to circulate the blood. Quitting reduces this risk by 50% at least.

Stroke risk: The increased blood pressure also increases the risk for stroke.

Peripheral vascular disease: Hardening of the arteries is caused or increased by smoking. Quitting improves circulation which improves your ability to exercise, and increases your overall survival rate.

Lung disease: Smoking constantly irritates the delicate lining of the airways and gives the voice a gravely quality. The constant irritation causes scarring, which causes lung disease. Quitting stops the further progression of chronic lung disease, and as the inflammation heals, lets you breathe easier.

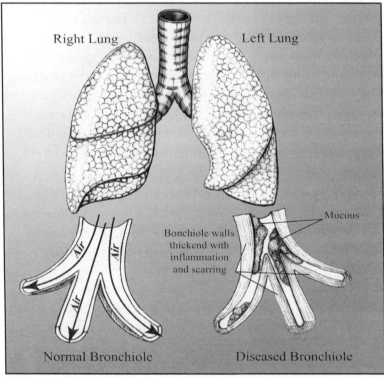

Figure 1. Lungs with normal bonchiole and a diseased bronchiole as a result of smoking

What are the benefits of quitting?

Less risk of heart, vascular, and lung disease are the major benefits of quitting smoking. No more smoker's cough and fewer respiratory infections lead to more productive days. Breathing is easier, and you will have more energy. There will be clean air for your family, as well as a clean smell at home and in your car. You will save money, and there will be no more burn holes in your clothes and upholstery. You breath will smell better and your complexion will take on a healthier color.

Is nicotine really addictive?

Nicotine has a powerful effect on the body, changing mood, alertness, and energy level. These effects are pleasing to the smoker and therefore reinforce the act of using tobacco. Over time, the body adapts to an expected level of nicotine in the system, and a "normal state" is achieved only when smoking routinely. Nicotine can be psychologically addicting as well. The tobacco user comes to depend on nicotine to cope with many feelings including stress, discomfort, anger, anxiety and loneliness. When nicotine is no longer available, the smoker may feel a great sense of loss or even panic that the "trusted friend" is gone.

What are the symptoms of nicotine withdrawal?

Here is a list of common nicotine withdrawal symptoms:
- Craving
- Irritability
- Insomnia
- Increased appetite
- Inability to concentrate
- Fatigue
- Constipation, gas, stomach pain
- Coughing

Withdrawal can last for several weeks to several months, with the symptoms the strongest in the first 1-4 days. These can be eased with Nicotine Replacement Products.

Aren't Nicotine Replacement Products as harmful as using tobacco?

No! They don't have all the tars and poisonous gasses that are found in cigarettes. They provide less nicotine than a smoker would get from cigarettes. And they are designed to get people off nicotine, not keep them addicted. Smokers who use some form of *Nicotine Replacement Product (NRP)* and participate in a behavior change program can double their chances of quitting for good.

How do I use Nicotine Replacement Products?

Nicotine Replacement Products quiet the urges from the nicotine receptors in the brain but lack the other feedback to the user, like handling, taste, smell, and other aspects of tobacco use that are pleasing to the user.

- *Nicotine patches* – available over-the-counter (without doctor's prescription) in 21, 14 and 7 mg strengths. They provide a constant, steady nicotine level to soften the urges throughout the day or night. They take effect slowly; so don't expect immediate relief from urges.
- *Nicotine gum or lozenges* – also over-the-counter in 2 or 4 mg strengths. These take effect within a few minutes and provide fairly fast relief. They can be used with the patch for intense urges that won't go away with deep breathing or distraction.
- *Nicotine inhaler* or *nose spray* – by prescription only. These are also fast-acting products.
- *Bupropion (Wellbutrin, Zyban) – non-nicotine prescription antidepressant* that works on the nicotine receptors of the brain to soften the urges to smoke.

CAUTION: Never use tobacco products while using nicotine replacement products, as serious health conditions can occur.

These nicotine replacement products can be weaned when the quitter is comfortable with their new tobacco-free lifestyle, usually in 2-3 months. Then the strength of the NRP should be gradually tapered. If you don't feel comfortable eliminating NRP after 3 months, consult your physician before continuing use.

What are some quitting strategies?

A *quit date* should be set within a couple of weeks of the decision to quit. Many tobacco users find *gradual reduction* helpful prior to their quit date. This is a method of reducing the number of cigarettes smoked per day or eliminating places or time of the day when you allow yourself to smoke. Some smokers switch brands to reduce the pleasure found in smoking. These are ways to practice quitting and build the quitter's confidence. The *abrupt cessation* is necessary to be successful. The *use of nicotine replacement products* makes this transition much more comfortable and increases your chance of success.

How do I resist the urges to smoke after I quit?

While NRP's are helpful, they are not a "magic pill." Other techniques that are helpful to resist the urge to smoke include:

- Breathe deeply
- Go for a walk
- Chew sugarless gum or eat sugarless hard candy
- Work with your hands: sew, knit, crochet, woodworking

- Chew on vegetable sticks
- Brush your teeth
- Squeeze a small rubber ball
- Drink plenty of water
- Work in the yard

Did we mention **deep breathing?** This is very important, as deep breathing is part of the relaxation smokers get from cigarettes. Keep breathing deeply – just lose the smoke!

Why is relaxation so important?

Since many tobacco users rely on tobacco for relaxation, new ways to relax and handle stress must be developed.

- **Relaxation:** Deep breathing, stretching, making time to be alone, or doing something with someone you enjoy.
- **Problem-solving:** Analyze a problem and work toward a solution.
- **Time management:** List short- and long-term goals, and schedule daily time according to priorities.

Additional tips:
- Take 5-minute breaks
- Do neck and shoulder rubs
- Engage in exercise
- Limit alcohol, sugar, salt, and caffeine
- Get plenty of sleep
- Talk to someone about your feelings

If I am not successful quitting on the first try, should I give up?

Of course not! Think about why you lapsed, and determine what you will do differently next time. Then make plans to get back on track ASAP. Remember, 25% of first time quitters have a lapse. Many quitters take 2-5 attempts before they make it for good. A lapse becomes a relapse if you give up trying!

Who should I choose for my support system, and why are they important?

You must make the decision to quit smoking for yourself, but you don't have to do it alone. Asking for others' help is a positive part of the process. The first people you may think of for support are family members. You must also consider people with whom you spend most of your day, possibly co-workers. Think also about friends and social contacts that will be willing to help. It will be very helpful if at least one of these support people is a former smoker. We all need suggestions, recognition and encouragement from others.

I have been using spit tobacco. Is it as harmful as smoking? How do I quit that?

Smokeless, or spit tobacco, users are also addicted to nicotine, with "normal" levels higher than smokers! The health risks include abrasion of the teeth, gum recession, bone loss around teeth, white pre-cancerous lesions in mouth, oral cancer and cardiovascular disease. Since tobacco juice is sometimes swallowed, digestive system cancers are also more common. Nicotine gum or lozenges are an effective substitute for spit tobacco.

I don't want to quit because I will gain weight. How do people avoid weight gain when they quit?

The average weight gain for quitters is 7-10 pounds. If you include a healthy lifestyle, with exercise and healthy eating as part of your plan, weight gain can be minimized. No matter what your weight is now, you will be healthier with a few extra pounds and without tobacco!

Nutrition as We Age
Elaine Guthrie, RD, LD/N

How important is good nutrition?

As we get older, we become more aware of the need to eat right to remain healthy and to feel good.

Benefits of nutritious eating include:
- Living a longer and healthier life
- Looking and feeling better
- A higher energy level
- Staying mentally sharp
- A positive outlook on life
- A strong immune system
- Being able to recover faster from illness
- Better able to perform daily activities to remain independent
- Ability to reach and maintain your proper weight
- A lower risk for obesity, diabetes, heart disease, cancer and high blood pressure

Health experts believe that poor eating habits increase our chances of having a chronic illness. The good news is that by making positive nutritional changes and making good nutrition a way of life, we can improve our lives.

What should I eat?

The 2005 **Dietary Guidelines for Americans** gives science-based advice on healthy food and physical activity choices.

These include:
- Eat a variety of foods within and among the basic food groups while not going over calorie needs.
- Control calorie intake to manage body weight.
- Be physically active every day.
- Increase daily intake of fruits and vegetables, whole grains, and nonfat or low-fat milk and milk products.
- Keep intake of saturated fat, trans fat and cholesterol low.
- Choose fiber-rich carbohydrates (fruits, vegetables, and whole grains) often and reduce intake of added sugar.
- Eat and prepare foods with little or no salt.
- If you drink alcoholic beverages, do so in moderation.
- Keep food safe to eat.

There are two eating plans that show you how to eat according to the new dietary guidelines.

USDA Food Guide (Pyramid)

Recommendations per day for a healthy diet for the average adult over the age of 50 years old include:
- *Grains (5-6 oz.)*
  1 ounce = 1 slice bread, 1 cup ready-to-eat cereal, ½ cup cooked cereal, cooked rice, or cooked pasta. Make half of your grains whole grain.
- *Vegetables (2-2 1/2 cups)*
  1 cup = raw or cooked vegetables, vegetable juice or 2 cups raw leafy greens.
- *Fruits (1 ½-2 cups)*
  1 cup = 1 cup fruit or 100% fruit juice or ½ cup dried fruit. Go easy on fruit juice.
- *Milk, yogurt and cheese (3 cups)*
  1 cup = 1 cup milk or yogurt, 1 ½ ounces natural cheese or 2 ounces processed cheese (includes milk-

based desserts such as pudding, ice cream and frozen yogurt.)

- *Meats and Beans (5-5 ½ oz.)*
  1 ounce = 1 oz. meat, poultry or fish, ¼ cup cooked dry beans, 1 egg, 1 tablespoon peanut butter, ½ oz. nuts or seeds.
- *Oils (5-6 teaspoons)*
- *Discretionary calories (130-265 calories)*
  Calories you can use for additional foods that are fat-free or low-fat and with no added sugars.

DASH Eating Plan (Dietary Approaches to Stop Hypertension)

Originally designed to prevent and treat hypertension, it too is a balanced eating plan. Based on consuming 2,000 calories a day, the DASH diet recommends:

- *7-8 servings of grains or grain products* to provide energy and fiber. This includes whole-wheat breads, cereals and oatmeal. One serving would equal 1 slice of bread, 1 oz. dry cereal, or ½ cup cooked rice or pasta.
- *4-5 servings of vegetables:* Vegetables are good sources of potassium, magnesium and fiber. A serving of vegetables is equivalent to 1 cup raw leafy vegetables, ½ cup cooked vegetable, or 6 oz. vegetable juice.
- *4-5 servings of fruits*: Fruits are also good sources of potassium, magnesium and fiber. A serving of fruits equals 1 medium fruit, ¼ cup dried fruit, ½ cup fresh, frozen, or canned fruit, or 6 oz. fruit juice.
- *2-3 servings of low-fat or non-fat dairy products* that provide calcium and protein. A serving of dairy equals 8 oz. milk, 1 cup yogurt, 1 ½ oz. cheese.
- *No more than 2 servings of meat, poultry, or fish:* These are good sources of protein and magnesium. A serving is 3 oz., which is the size of a deck of cards.

131

- *4-5 servings of nuts, seeds, or dry beans:* These are good sources of energy, magnesium, potassium, protein and fiber. A serving is 1/3 cup nuts, 2 tbsp. seeds, and ½ cup cooked dry beans.
- *1-3 servings of fats and oils:* A serving equals 1 tsp. soft margarine, 1 tbsp. low-fat mayonnaise, 2 tbsp. light salad dressing, or 1 tsp. vegetable oil.
- *5 sweets per week:* A serving of sweets is equal to 1 tbsp. sugar, jelly, or jam, or 8 oz. lemonade.

Some other tips:
- Make small changes over time.
- Try foods you haven't tried before.
- Enjoy all foods in moderation.

Do I need to cut back on calories?

As you get older, your body needs fewer calories because it tends to burn fewer calories due to losing muscle and gaining fat. Muscle burns more calories than fat. Also, you may not be as physically active as you used to be.

You need to balance calories from foods and beverages with the calories you burn through exercise. If you go over your calories from food and beverages, you will gain weight. If you take in fewer calories, you will lose weight.

You can keep from losing muscle and maintain a healthy body weight by doing both aerobic and strength-training exercises. Also, make sure you are consuming a well-balanced diet with adequate protein.

Even though your body requires fewer calories, the needs for protein, vitamins and minerals stay the same or increase. Eat a variety of foods high in nutrients and moderate to low in calories. These include:

- Lean protein, such as lean meat, fish or poultry
- Low-fat dairy
- Grains
- Fruits and vegetables

There are some special considerations.

Overweight

Over ½ of older Americans are overweight and 1/3 are obese due to:
- Overeating
- Poor food choices
- Inactivity

Being overweight increases your risk for:
- Diabetes
- Heart disease
- Osteoarthritis (wearing away of the joints)

To help lose weight:
- Never skip a meal.
- Watch portion sizes.
- Avoid empty calorie foods such as regular soda pop, excessive sweets, and hidden fats; they contain a lot of calories, but little nutrition.
- Keep a food record.
- Exercise on a regular basis.

Underweight
To help gain weight:
- Eat four to six smaller meals a day.
- Drink milk, juice or shakes more often than coffee, tea, or diet sodas.
- Snack on higher-calorie foods such as peanut butter and crackers or dried fruit.

- Use milk instead of water when preparing hot cereal or soup.
- Use extra margarine on vegetables, breads, hot cereal, rice or noodles, and add to soup.
- Try a nutritional supplement drink.

Determine your daily calorie needs from the USDA chart.

Calorie Range

Children	Sedentary		Active
2-3 Years	1,000	→	1,400
Females			
4-8 Years	1,200	→	1,800
9-13	1,600	→	2,200
14-18	1,800	→	2,400
19-30	2,000	→	2,400
31-50	1,800	→	2,200
51+	1,600	→	2,200
Males			
4-8 Years	1,400	→	2,000
9-13	1,800	→	2,600
14-18	2,200	→	3,200
19-30	2,400	→	3,000
31-50	2,200	→	3,000
51+	2,000	→	2,800

Sedentary means a lifestyle that includes only the light physical activity associated with typical day-to-day life.

Active means a lifestyle that includes physical activity equivalent to walking more than 3 miles per day at 3 to 4 miles per hour, in addition to the light physical activity associated with typical day-to-day life.

U.S. Department of Agriculture
Center for Nutrition Policy and Promotion
April 2005

How much fiber should I be eating?

According to the *American Dietetic Association*, the recommended daily allowance of *dietary fiber* for men is 30-38 grams per day and for women is 21-25 grams, of which 5-10 grams of fiber should be soluble. Fiber is important for a healthy heart and digestive system.

There are two types of *fiber*: *insoluble* and *soluble*. Insoluble fiber is the roughage we need to prevent constipation, *diverticulosis* (pouches in the lining of the large intestine that can become inflamed, be very painful, and lead to more serious problems), *gallstones* and *colon cancer*. It is found in whole grains, vegetables, wheat bran, nuts, and beans. Whole grains also contain *phytochemicals (plant chemicals)* that reduce the risk of heart disease.

Soluble fiber has been shown to reduce *LDL cholesterol ("bad cholesterol") levels*. It attaches itself to cholesterol in your gut and prevents it from being absorbed into your bloodstream. Good sources of soluble fiber are oats, barley, beans, lentils, peas, nuts, seeds, apples, the grain psyllium, as well as other fruits and vegetables. A number of studies have shown that oats may also lower blood pressure. Foods that contain 2-4 grams of soluble fiber are:

- 1 ½ cups cooked oatmeal
- ½ cup cooked dried beans
- 1 piece of citrus fruit or pear
- ½ cup Brussels sprouts
- ½ cup yogurt with fiber

A high-fiber diet can also help keep blood sugars in check and help you lose weight. The best source of fiber is from food, rather than from dietary supplements. When increasing the amount of fiber in your diet, add it gradually, as too much too soon can cause cramping and bloating. Also, because added fiber requires added liquids, make sure you are drinking adequate amounts of fluids.

How much water should I drink?
Try to drink 6 to 8 eight-ounce glasses of water a day, unless you have been told to drink less by your health care provider. Milk and juice can count toward your daily amount of water. Coffee, tea and alcoholic beverages do not count because they draw fluid out of the body.

Water is needed for the following reasons:
- Cells and organs depend on water to function.
- It is a major part of saliva and the fluid around the joints.
- It carries nutrients to all body cells.
- Water helps the kidneys remove waste products from the body.
- It may help to prevent kidney stones.
- Water keeps fiber moving in the body and adds bulk to stools to prevent constipation.

As we age, we lose some of our sense of thirst and therefore feel less thirsty; however, our bodies still need the same amount of water. Total body water decreases with age from 60% to 50%, so we have less supply. Be careful not to become dehydrated. Be sure to drink additional water in times of sickness with vomiting or diarrhea and with heavy sweating.

Do I need a multivitamin/mineral supplement?
Food is the best way to get the vitamins, minerals and other nutrients your body needs. However, there are times when you might need a *vitamin/mineral supplement*. These include:
- Falling short of eating the recommended number of

servings from the food guide pyramid or the DASH eating plan.
- Being on a very low-calorie weight-loss diet or a vegetarian diet.
- Unable to drink milk or eat cheese and yogurt.
- Having a poor appetite and not eating as much as you should.

Make sure to check the label and look for a supplement that does not contain more than 100% of the *Daily Value (DV)*. Taking more than 100% of certain vitamins and minerals can harm your health. For example, too much vitamin A can cause liver damage. Also, large amounts can interfere with how your medications work.

The 2005 **Dietary Guidelines** has two recommendations concerning vitamins for people over the age of 50.

1. *Everyone over 50 years old should consume at least 2.4 micrograms of vitamin B-12 per day from fortified foods or a B-12 supplement.* Many people this age do not secrete enough stomach acid to be able to absorb the natural B-12 in food. Vitamin B-12 is needed to develop normal red blood cells and maintain healthy nerve cells. A deficiency can cause *pernicious anemia,* of which one symptom may be *dementia.* Some older people diagnosed with dementia actually have a vitamin B-12 deficiency which can be easily treated.

2. *Older adults should consume extra vitamin D fortified foods and/or supplements.* The *Dietary Reference Intakes* recommends 400 IU for ages 50-70 and 600 IU for over 70 years old. As we age we lose the ability to absorb the vitamin D from sunlight due to thinning skin and less time spent in the sun.

Vitamin D maintains normal levels of calcium and phosphorus in the body to help form strong bones.

Calcium also becomes more important as we age to help improve bone density and to prevent fractures. The *National Institute of Health* recommends adults over the age of 50 should get 1200 mg a day and men over the age of 65 as well as post-menopausal women not on bone-building drugs should aim for 1500 mg calcium a day. Having enough vitamin D helps the body to absorb calcium. Calcium may also help to keep blood pressure low and play a role in preventing colon cancer. If you are not a milk drinker and do not eat many dairy products, you will need to take supplements that contain *calcium carbonate* or *calcium citrate*. Note, however, that calcium carbonate supplements may cause you to be constipated.

Should I be drinking a nutritional supplement?

Despite the TV ads that make drinking *liquid nutritional supplements* look fashionable, they are unnecessary unless you are unable to meet your nutrition needs from food. These times may include:

- Recovering from sickness or surgery
- Poor appetite resulting in weight loss
- Needing a convenient meal replacement

There are a variety of helpful commercial supplements in many flavors. They can resemble a thin milkshake or a fruit drink and contain a balance of vitamins, minerals, protein, and calories. Most are lactose-free. Supplements are also available in bars and puddings.

What kind of diet should I follow if I have a chronic health condition?

Diabetes

Diabetes is a condition in which your body does not make enough of a hormone called *insulin* or is unable to use the insulin you do have effectively. Insulin allows your cells to absorb sugar in your blood to be used for energy or be stored for a later use. When *blood sugar (glucose)* is not able to get into our cells, it builds up in the bloodstream or spills over into our urine. Without energy, we cannot perform our daily activities. When not controlled, diabetes can lead to long-term health problems such as *heart disease*, *strokes*, *poor circulation*, *vision loss* and *kidney failure*.

It is important to eat a well-balanced meal based on the calorie level that is right for you. Also, carbohydrates (grains, fruits, vegetables, milk and sweets) should be eaten in a consistent manner. Your dietitian or health care provider can recommend appropriate carbohydrate amounts for you. Counting carbohydrates in the foods you eat can help make control of your blood glucose levels easier and give you more flexibility in making food choices. Eat the same number of carbohydrates at each meal and for snacks. You will also be watching meat and meat substitutes as well as fat. Generally, you will need no more than 6 ounces of meat or meat substitutes a day and 3-5 servings of fat a day.

Some helpful suggestions include:
- Never skip meals
- Eat at about the same time every day, with meals about 4-5 hours apart
- Eat a variety of foods
- Make sure to eat foods high in fiber; fiber helps to control blood sugar
- Avoid fried foods

- Watch portion sizes especially when eating out
- Monitor your weight; losing only 10 pounds can improve blood sugars in Type 2 diabetes
- Exercise every day
- Watch out for sugar-free candies; they still contain calories and/or sugar alcohols, which can raise blood sugar
- Use the nutrition facts on the food label to see how much carbohydrate is in a serving

Hypercholesterolemia (High Cholesterol)
Cholesterol is a waxy, fatty substance that can harden arteries in our heart, neck or kidneys if we have high levels in our blood.

Ways to help lower cholesterol include:
- Limit total fat eaten in one day to approximately 40 grams for a woman and 50 grams for a man
- Decrease *saturated fat*. Saturated fats come mainly from foods of animal origin such as butter, fatty meats, full-fat dairy products and cheese. Saturated fats increase low-density lipoprotein (LDL), or the bad cholesterol.
- Eat primarily unsaturated fat. There are two types of unsaturated fats: monounsaturated and polyunsaturated. *Monounsaturated fats* include olive and canola oil, avocados and nuts. Monounsaturated fats help to lower LDL cholesterol without lowering our good cholesterol (HDL). *Polyunsaturated fats* include omega-3 and omega-6 fatty acids. *Omega-3 fatty acids* include *flaxseed* and *fish oils* that are found in cold-water fish. Omega-6 fatty acids include the vegetable oils (corn, safflower, soybean and sunflower). Using polyunsaturated fats in place of saturated fat in the diet helps to lower LDL and raise HDL cholesterol.

- Limit intake of foods with high cholesterol content such as egg yolks (3 a week) and organ meats.
- Avoid *trans fats*. Trans-fatty acids are made through a process called *hydrogenation*, which changes a liquid fat to a solid one. Trans fats are found in many store-bought baked goods and convenience foods, as well as in some margarines. This type of fat raises LDL cholesterol. Read labels to learn how much trans fat is in the food.
- Eat *soluble fiber*. Soluble fiber has been shown to reduce LDL cholesterol. Good sources of soluble fiber are *oats, barley, beans, lentils, peas, nuts, seeds, apples,* the grain *psyllium*, as well as other fruits and vegetables.
- Increase your intake of fruits and vegetables to obtain *phytochemicals* (plant chemicals that fight heart disease).
- Lose weight if needed. Small amounts of *weight loss* can lower LDL cholesterol.

Hypertriglyceridemia (High triglycerides)
Triglycerides are another type of fat found in the blood. Triglycerides should be less than 150 mg/dl. If they are high, they can be a risk factor for heart disease, more in women than men.

Ways to help lower triglycerides include:
- Follow a diet low in saturated fat and cholesterol.
- Control your weight.
- Increase physical activity.
- Restrict alcohol.
- Start eating foods high in omega-3 fatty acids, such as sardines, salmon, mackerel, tuna, swordfish, herring and rainbow trout twice a week.
- Try using ground flaxseed, 1-2 tbsp a day, in cereals, yogurt, fruit juice or salads. Flaxseed also contains

141

omega-3 fatty acids, which have been shown to lower triglycerides.

Hypertension (High blood pressure)

High blood pressure is one of the controllable risk factors for strokes, heart attacks and heart failure. A blood pressure higher than 120 over 80 needs to be lowered. When blood pressure is too high, the heart is working harder than it should. Once you develop high blood pressure it is likely that it will be a lifetime problem.

High blood pressure can be controlled or even prevented by the following steps:
- Lose weight if you need to.
- Be physically active.
- Follow a healthy eating plan such as the USDA food guide pyramid or the DASH eating plan.
- Choose foods lower in salt and sodium; limit cured or smoked meat, vegetables in a brine solution such as pickles or olives, salty snacks, canned and processed foods; season foods with herbs and spices, lemon juice, flavored vinegars.
- Limit alcohol.

Osteoporosis (Brittle-bone disease)

Osteoporosis is a disease in which bones weaken gradually to the point that they can fracture under normal use. Both men and women can develop this disease. Beginning in our 30's and 40's, we start to lose bone mass. Women will lose bone mass rapidly in the first 5 to 10 years after menopause. As we age, bones become thinner because they are losing calcium faster than they gain it. We can slow down the rate at which our bones lose calcium by:
- **Eating calcium-rich foods such as milk, cheese and yogurt:** Adults over the age of 50 need 1200 mg. of calcium a day and men over the age of 65 and

post-menopausal women not on bone-building drugs should have 1500 mg calcium.

- **Consuming extra vitamin D fortified foods and/or supplements:** 400 IU vitamin D for ages 50-70 and 600 IU for over 70 years old.
- **Doing weight-bearing exercise** (walking, aerobic exercise).
- **Not consuming excess caffeine, sodium, phosphorus and alcohol.**

Are there foods that can help prevent diseases?

Phytochemicals (natural chemicals found in plants) are associated with the prevention and/or treatment of at least 4 of the leading causes of death in the United States: cancer, heart disease, diabetes and hypertension. There are over 900 different phytochemicals found in fruits, vegetables, whole grains, nuts, seeds and herbal seasonings. They are substances that plants produce to protect themselves against viruses, bacteria, and fungi. It is important to eat a variety of whole foods and not extracts or supplements. Also, there are other foods that contain vitamins, minerals, or nutrients that can help prevent diseases.

The top twelve disease-fighting foods include:
- ***Beans:*** Beans lower the risk of developing breast, colon and prostate cancer and ½ cup a day can lower cholesterol by 10%.
- ***Berries:*** Blueberries may help keep our minds sharp, lessen brain damage from strokes, reduce the buildup of LDL cholesterol in our arteries, and may reduce the effects of Alzheimer's disease or dementia. Strawberries, raspberries and blackberries contain anti-cancer substances.
- ***Cabbage:*** A phytochemical in cabbage makes cells rid themselves of cancerous substances. Eating

cabbage may help protect against breast, lung, stomach, and colon cancers.

- ***Citrus fruits:*** Citrus fruits are high in vitamin C, which helps your body fight cancers (lung, cervical, esophagus and stomach). Grapefruit may also reduce the risk of macular degeneration.
- ***Cold-water fish:*** Cold-water fish (sardines, salmon, mackerel, tuna, swordfish, and herring) contain omega-3 fatty acids that lower the risk for heart attack, hypertension, and stroke. A higher intake of omega-3s also helps maintain your bone mass. It is better to eat wild salmon and avoid eating the skin as farm-raised salmon and skin may contain cancer-causing compounds.
- ***Flaxseed:*** 1-2 tbsp. ground flaxseed a day reduces the risk of heart disease as well as cancer.
- ***Garlic:*** Garlic lowers cholesterol and blood pressure and reduces the risk for colon and possibly stomach cancer.
- ***Nuts:*** Nuts can help prevent heart disease by lowering LDL cholesterol and keeping arteries more elastic.
- ***Tea:*** Drinking white, green, oolong or black teas – ***not*** herbal teas – on a regular basis may protect arteries from plaque buildup and reduce risk of cancer. If you are taking coumadin, you should not drink green or herbal teas.
- ***Tomatoes:*** Tomatoes are high in vitamin C and rich in the phytochemical ***lycopene***, which may lower LDL cholesterol and prevent cancer growth.
- ***Whole grains:*** Research shows that eating three daily servings of whole grains can reduce the risk of heart disease by 25 to 36 percent, stroke by 37 percent, and type 2 diabetes by 21 to 27 percent.
- ***Yogurt:*** Yogurt contains the friendly bacteria (active) that help fight illness or disease.

Do I need to avoid certain foods because of the medications I take?

- *Aspirin* and *ibuprofen* should be taken with meals because they can irritate an empty stomach.

- Do not eat *dairy foods* or take a *calcium supplement* at the same time you take the antibiotic *tetracycline* or its derivatives. Wait two hours before having any calcium-containing food or supplement because calcium can block the absorption of the drug.

- While on *coumadin*, eat a predictable and consistent amount of foods high in *Vitamin K* such as green vegetables, liver and soybean oil. Vitamin K can make the blood clot faster. Avoid *alcohol*.

- If you are taking an antidepressant that is a *monoamine oxidase inhibitor (MAO)*, you need to avoid foods high in *tyramine*. These include aged cheese, caviar, liver, canned figs, soy sauce, sauerkraut, fava beans (Italian), yeasts, yogurt, red wine, and beer. Avoid smoked or pickled meat, poultry, and fish. Do not eat dried fruit, bananas, avocados, raspberries, or very ripe fruit. Avoid excessive amounts of caffeine. Eating these foods while on the medication could lead to a deadly change in blood pressure.

- If you are on a *gout medication* such as *Allopurinol*, it is important to drink at least 10-12 glasses of *water* a day and to avoid *alcohol*.

- *Grapefruit juice* changes the way the body processes some medications such as certain cholesterol-lowering drugs and high blood pressure medicines. It increases the absorption rate, which may lead to toxic levels of these drugs.

- *Potassium-containing salt substitutes* can interact with *"water" pills* or *blood pressure medicines* to increase blood potassium levels. This can cause

145

nausea, vomiting, muscle cramps, diarrhea, weakness and cardiac arrest.

What can I do if I have problems eating?
No appetite
Suggestions:

- Check with your doctor to see if your lack of appetite is due to any of the medicines you take.
- Eat several small meals.
- Cold or room-temperature meals may be more appealing.
- Make your food look and taste good; include some colorful foods on your plate and dress your table with a colorful place mat or flower; add spices or herbs to your food for flavor.
- Do regular moderate exercise.
- If possible, eat with family and friends or go to a group senior meal service.
- A liquid nutritional supplement may be needed.

Loss of taste and smell
Situation: At around the age of 60, we lose some of our ability to taste and smell; at 75, we will have half as many taste buds as we did at age 30.

- Increase the flavor of your food by adding flavor enhancers instead of salt and fat, such as: olive oil, vinegar, garlic, onions, spices, herbs, powdered butter flavorings, and vanilla or almond extracts to desserts
- Serve warm, not overly hot, foods
- Chew slowly to allow odors to reach your nose

Dry mouth
Situation: Due to changes in our digestive system, our bodies make less saliva.

Suggestions:

- Eating or drinking tart foods such as citrus fruits, lemonade or cranberry juice will stimulate saliva production in your mouth
- Sugar-free gum or hard candy can also help produce saliva
- Increase moisture in your food by adding soup, gravy, sauces, or milk
- If dryness is severe, you may benefit from artificial saliva

Can't chew

Situation: It may be hard for you to chew food due to loose teeth, poorly fitting dentures or a sore mouth from gum disease or a medication reaction.

Suggestions:

- Change the texture of your food as needed (soft, ground, pureed, or liquid)
- Take small bites
- Eat moist foods such as casseroles
- Drink liquids with your meals to make chewing easier

Upset stomach

Situation: As we age, we produce less stomach acid and it is harder for our bodies to digest food. This can result in bloating, heartburn, and constipation.

Suggestions:

- Eat small, frequent meals
- Drink lots of fluids
- Eat more fiber
- Take the time to eat slowly and to chew your food well

Swallowing difficulties
Suggestions:

- Discuss with your doctor; the texture of your food may need to be changed and/or you may need to be evaluated by a speech therapist
- Slow down – foods or beverages that are swallowed too fast can result in dangerous choking
- When food, drink, or saliva from your mouth goes into your lungs it can cause an infection, called ***aspiration pneumonia***

Should I be concerned with food safety?

As you lose your sense of taste, smell and possibly eyesight, you may not always be able to tell if foods have gone bad. **If in doubt, throw it out.** You may want to label foods in the refrigerator with the date you store it to keep yourself from eating foods that are no longer fresh.

Also, your immune system may not be as strong and you are at a higher risk for illness.

Other guidelines to prevent food-borne illness include:

- Always clean your hands, food contact surfaces, and fruits and vegetables.
- Do not wash or rinse meat and poultry.
- Keep raw, cooked and ready-to-eat foods separate while shopping, preparing, or storing foods.
- Make sure your refrigerator temperature stays below 40 degrees.
- Change dish rags, sponges and dish towels often.
- Cook foods to a safe temperature to kill microorganisms – certain foods such as eggs, pork, fish, shellfish, poultry, and hot dogs need to be well-cooked to prevent disease.
- Refrigerate perishable foods promptly after you

purchase them.
- Defrost your foods in the refrigerator or in the microwave, never on the countertop.
- Avoid raw (unpasteurized) milk or milk products, unpasteurized juices or raw sprouts.
- Never let food sit at the table for more than 2 hours, or 1 hour in hot weather. Refrigerate leftovers promptly and eat within 3 or 4 days. Cool hot food items first before putting into the refrigerator for storage.

How should I plan meals?
- Plan one to two weeks at a time.
- Include an entree, starch or bread, vegetable or salad, and a fruit or dessert for lunch and/or supper.
- Consider special dietary needs.
- Make a grocery list of what you need; be sure to check your supply of staples like flour, sugar, rice, and cereal, as well as any canned or frozen foods on hand.
- Check grocery store ads for specials and go through your coupons.
- Look at cookbooks for recipe ideas and write down any ingredients you will need.
- Include planned leftovers for other meals.

What should I consider when shopping for food?
- Be sure to bring your grocery list, coupons, eyeglasses and calculator.
- Think about how much of a product you will use — larger sizes are not always cheaper, especially if you end up throwing some of it away.
- Consider using store and generic brands for good food at a lower price.
- Stock up on sale items or specials only if you will use

them at a later date.
- Avoid impulse buying— try to stick to your list; foods bought on impulse are often high in calories with little nutritional value.
- Put refrigerated or frozen foods in your cart last.
- Check the food labels to help you choose a good diet.

What are some tips for healthy cooking?
- Cook foods to a safe temperature.
- Fully cook meat, fish, and poultry, but don't overcook your vegetables.
- Prepare foods with little or no salt.
- Bake, barbecue, steam, boil or microwave foods instead of frying.
- Use two egg whites in a recipe in place of a whole egg.
- Rinse cooked ground beef in a strainer with hot water before adding to a recipe.
- Try using spices and herbs to flavor your foods.
- Cook ahead and freeze portions to have healthy and easy meals for when you don't feel like cooking.
- It's ok to use packaged, cut-up vegetables and pre-washed, pre-cut salad greens.
- Use leftover meats and vegetables in casseroles, soups, or omelets.

What can I do to eat healthy if I don't cook?
- Buy prepared foods and dinners that contain less sodium and fat and heat them in the oven or microwave.
- Take advantage of senior meal programs.
- Hire a homemaker to shop and prepare meals for you.
- Consider the Meals on Wheels program if you are homebound and/or disabled or unable to provide meals for yourself. Meals on Wheels provide 1-2

balanced meals delivered to your home daily for a small fee.

What are some guidelines for healthy eating at restaurants?

- Watch portion sizes. Restaurants generally serve double or triple the amount of food you actually need. Order smaller portions if possible or take half of your meal home to reheat for another day.
- Share a meal or parts of a meal such as an entree, appetizer, or dessert with your dining partner.
- Have an appetizer instead of a main course.
- Avoid buffets. Buffets encourage overeating and make it easy to consume a high fat meal.
- Choose foods from a light menu or those marked as healthy choices.
- Order main courses that are baked, broiled, roasted, poached, or steamed.
- Choose salads with light dressings and fruit.
- Ask for vegetables and main dishes without sauces.
- Ask to have foods made in a more healthy way.
- Balance the meals you eat in restaurants with the foods you eat at home to meet your nutritional needs.

Remember: It's never too late to improve the way you eat. It all starts by what you put on your plate!

Chapter 12

The Disease of Obesity
Denise Strathdee, RD, LD, LMHC

How serious is the disease of obesity?

Obesity is an epidemic in the United States. In 1999-2002, 65 percent of adults age 20-74 were overweight and 31 percent were obese. Between 1988-94 and 1999-2002, obesity increased from 31 to 39 percent in adults 55-64 years of age. Overweight and obesity affect males and females, all ages, all racial and ethnic groups, all educational levels and all smoking levels. Obesity increases a person's risk for developing chronic diseases such as diabetes, high blood pressure, stroke, heart disease and some forms of cancer. The total costs attributed to obesity-related diseases approach $100 billion annually in the United States.

Americans spend over $30 billion yearly on dieting and weight-loss efforts, often to end up heavier, more discouraged and in worse health than when they started. What can a person do to control his or her weight and decrease health risks?

What are the health risks of obesity?

Obesity increases the risk of developing many diseases which negatively affect the length and quality of life. These include:
- Type 2 diabetes
- High blood pressure
- Elevated blood fats
- Cardiovascular disease
- Stroke
- Gallbladder disease
- Esophageal reflux disease
- Asthma

- Sleep apnea
- Gout
- Osteoarthritis
- Certain cancers
- Gynecological abnormalities
- Stress incontinence

Being overweight or obese can result in social stigmatization.

How do I know if I'm overweight or obese?

A person who is overweight is carrying an excess of body weight which includes muscle, bone, fat and water. Individuals who are very athletic may technically be overweight, but that is due to having extra muscle, not fat.

A person who is obese has excess body fat. We all need some body fat for insulation, energy storage, hormone production and other bodily functions. Males generally have less body fat than females and more muscle and bone. Males with more than 25 percent body fat and females with more than 30 percent body fat are considered obese.

The body mass index (BMI) is the standard used by health care providers to determine if a person is at a healthy weight, overweight or obese. The BMI uses a formula based on a person's height and weight. A BMI of 25-29.9 indicates a person is overweight. A BMI of 30-39.9 is considered obese. A BMI of 40 or more is considered morbidly obese. As the BMI goes up, risks of developing health problems increase.

It is also known that where a person carries fat on his or her body can increase one's risk of developing obesity-related health problems. Carrying too much fat around the waist increases disease risk. Males with a waist measurement of 40 inches or more and females with a waist measurement of 35

154

inches or more are at higher disease risk.

What causes obesity?

The disease of obesity is chronic and complex. There are several factors that may play a role in developing obesity.

While heredity may predispose a person to developing obesity, our genes alone do not automatically make us obese. The way we live – what we eat, how much we eat and how physically active we are – play key roles in whether we become obese. Our society consumes many high-fat, high-sugar foods and beverages. We say "super-size me" to get more value for our dollar, but in doing so, we eat more calories, fat, sodium, and sugar than our bodies need. We tend to be less active than past generations. Ironically, although we have more conveniences, we have less free time. Most Americans do not get enough exercise.

Emotional factors may affect our eating behavior. People often eat in response to negative feelings, such as anger, anxiety, boredom, depression, loneliness or stress. In these instances, food is used as a coping mechanism. While eating distracts us from the uncomfortable feeling temporarily, it does not make the situation that resulted in the negative feeling go away, so the negative feeling returns, along with guilt due to eating, and a cycle occurs.

Chronic dieting leads to obesity by producing physical and emotional deprivation. This typically results in *binge eating*. It is estimated that as many as one-third to one-half of people seeking medical services for weight loss have problems with binge eating. Binge eating is defined as eating amounts of food larger than what most people would eat within a two-hour period and feeling a loss of control over eating. People who binge-eat usually eat until they feel uncomfortably full, eat in secret and feel guilty after the episode. They typically have low self-esteem and may also be depressed. Addressing underlying emotional or psychological issues affecting eating behavior with a qualified health professional is important to regain control and optimize health and well-being.

There are some medical conditions that can cause weight gain or lead to obesity if untreated, such as hypothyroidism. Some medications, such as steroids and certain antidepressants, can result in weight gain.

Why is it so hard to lose weight and keep it off?

Our body has a *regulatory* or *set point weight* at which it is comfortable and fights to maintain. We can starve our bodies for a while and lose weight, but when we are once again allowed to eat without restriction, our bodies will make up for what we've missed by eating more, until we return to our former weight. Over time, with repeated cycles of dieting, we actually gain back more weight than we lost. In order to lose weight and keep it off, we have to change our regulatory or set point weight. The best way to do this is by a modest decrease in what we eat and daily exercise which increases the energy we burn.

Also, as we age, we tend to lose muscle tissue in our bodies and deposit fat around our internal organs. Our *metabolism*, or the rate at which we burn calories for energy, drops sharply after age 50. Our metabolism may drop as much as 30 percent throughout our life. This decreases our need for calories. If a person continues eating the same amount as he or she did when younger, that person will gradually gain weight.

Hormonal changes during perimenopause and menopause affect fat storage in the body. It is natural for women to gain

156

approximately 5 pounds of abdominal fat during menopause. Gaining an excess of abdominal fat, however, is not healthy because it is associated with increased risk of diabetes and heart disease.

What is the difference between physical hunger, "head" hunger, and emotional hunger?

When a person is *physically hungry*, his or her body usually sends signals, such as the stomach feeling empty or growling, slight fatigue, or perhaps a decrease in mental concentration or focus.

"Head" hunger does not involve these signals. Instead, it is the person's mind telling him or her it is time to eat based on the clock, because others are eating, or because the mind has been triggered by various cues to think it's time to eat. Examples of triggers include visual triggers, such as seeing food commercials on television, having candy in a bowl on your desk or seeing foods in the grocery store. Walking past a bakery and smelling pastries baking may trigger a desire to eat, although true physical hunger is not present.

Emotional hunger is usually in response to negative feelings such as anger, anxiety, boredom, depression, loneliness or stress. Eating is a way to distract from uncomfortable feelings. Some people eat when they feel happy or in a celebratory mood.

It is important to recognize what type of hunger one is experiencing in order to decide if eating is appropriate or not. Feeding "head" hunger results in developing an association between the trigger and eating which becomes a challenge to break. Emotional hunger is never truly satisfied by eating, as it represents a deeper need.

How can I increase my awareness of my hungers?

Ask yourself:

1) Is my body giving me physical signals that it's hungry? Has it been a few hours since I've last eaten? *(physical hunger)*

2) If I've eaten within the last 2 hours, is there something I'm seeing or smelling that is resulting in me thinking of eating? If I were not seeing or smelling these foods, would I be thinking about eating? *("head" hunger)*

3) Are others around me eating? Does the clock say it's time to eat, regardless of how I feel physically? *("head" hunger)*

4) Am I in a vulnerable state with my feelings right now? What am I feeling? It is important to identify feelings and "sit with them" versus trying to distract away from them. What is my need right now? Can I more effectively meet that need without turning to food as a coping mechanism? *(emotional hunger)*

What are key components of weight loss and weight management?

The emphasis is on *lifestyle changes*. These are changes that are made gradually but sustained, versus "going on" and "going off" a diet. They involve changing the way one thinks about food and eating. Accountability and support are important in order to sustain change. Key components are: *goal setting*, *nutrition*, *physical activity* and *behavioral changes*. We will discuss each as a separate category.

Goal setting

Three important goals for weight management are:

    a) Preventing further weight gain
    b) Producing weight loss
    c) Maintaining weight loss

Goal setting is important so you know where you are headed. Make sure your goals are reasonable. Too often, people expect to change everything overnight and end up frustrated, believing they can never change. Losing 10 percent of your current body weight (i.e., 15 lbs. if you currently weigh 150 lbs.) over 6 months can be enough to positively impact your health.

A reasonable weight loss goal would be 2-4 pounds per month. Start by changing one pattern or one food choice at a time. Write down your daily and weekly goals, and put them in a visible place where you will see them often. Tell someone else what your goals are. Give him or her permission to ask you about your progress. Give yourself a non-food reward when you meet your weekly or monthly goals. This helps you stay motivated.

Nutrition

What you eat is extremely important in how you think, feel and act. Food is your fuel. Too much or the wrong balance results in less than peak performance.

Healthy intake guidelines include:
    a) Eat at regular intervals throughout the day. Do not skip meals.
    b) Choose low-fat foods, grilled or baked rather than breaded or fried. Choose low-fat and fat-free dairy products. Do not add high-fat sauces or gravy.
    c) Some fat is necessary in the diet, but it should be small amounts of nuts or oils, such as walnuts, canola oil or olive oil, and omega-3 fats, found in such food as salmon. Avoid trans fats in packaged foods and saturated fats in animal products.
    d) Choose foods and beverages without a lot of

added sugar. Be careful of fruit juice – even though it is "natural," it is still high in sugar. Limit to ½ cup daily, or enjoy a piece of fresh fruit – the fiber will help you stay satisfied longer.

e) Limit alcohol.

f) Watch portions. No second helpings. Use smaller plates and bowls. Reduce portions by one-fourth to one-third.

g) Get plenty of fiber. Choose 100% whole grains, vegetables, and fruits.

h) Drink plenty of water, at least 6 – 8 cups daily.

i) Eat slowly, taking 20-30 minutes to finish a meal.

j) Eat mindfully, enjoying each bite. You will feel more satisfied when you're finished eating.

The following links from the United States Department of Agriculture can help you determine the appropriate number of calories to aim for daily, based upon your level of physical activity. The chart entitled "Food Intake Patterns" suggests the amounts of food to have daily from each food group based on your specific calorie needs. A week of sample menus based on 2000 calories daily is provided:

http://www.mypyramid.gov/downloads/MyPyramid_
Calorie_Levels.pdf
http://www.mypyramid.gov/downloads/sample_menu.pdf

Physical activity

Being physically active is a critical component of weight loss and weight maintenance, along with a reduced calorie intake. Often those who are overweight or obese have initial physical limitations which impact what kind of physical activity they can do and how long they can perform the activity. It is important to consult with your health professional to determine the best plan for you. Starting slowly and building slowly insure the best chances of avoiding injury and sticking with it. Building activity into each day can be done through deliberate exercise, such as walking for a certain length of time, and also by such strategies as parking further from a store in a parking lot or taking stairs instead of the elevator. It is recommended that adults set a long-term goal of performing at least 30 minutes or more of moderate-intensity physical activity on most, and preferably all, days of the week.

Behavioral changes
1) Self-monitoring of food intake, eating patterns, and weight

Start by keeping a detailed food diary for at least 1 week. Jot down everything you eat and drink, including amounts, the time of day and what you are doing when you eat. (See Table on page 160 for a sample food diary.)

After one week, look to see what patterns you notice. For instance, the person in this sample diary eats very little until 3 PM, and then consumes larger portions of higher-calorie foods from 3 PM – 9 PM. It is not surprising that this person would feel very hungry by supper and would overeat. Consuming multiple servings of caffeine throughout the day results in energy highs and lows. When a person feels tired, he or she may try to boost energy by eating, typically something with sugar that gives an immediate rise in energy, but this is not lasting. Notice that even though this person felt overly full after supper, he or she ate again later, likely triggered by watching television and feeling bored. This is the type of information one can obtain by self-monitoring.

Continuing food records, as well as recording physical activity, is important to stay on track as changes are made and continue progress.

It is a good idea to weigh yourself no more than once weekly, at the same time of day, on the same scale,

Table 1. Sample food diary

Day	Time	Food/ beverage	Amount	Activity	How I feel
Mon	6:30	Coffee, black & plain bagel	1 cup 1	Hurrying for work	Tired
Mon	10:30	Coffee, black	1 cup	Break	Tired
Mon	12:00	Light yogurt, apple, ice tea	1 carton 1 meduim 12 oz.	Eating with co-workers	Hungry
Mon	3:00	Candy bar	1	Working at desk	Stressed
Mon	6:00	Sausage pizza, diet pop	5 pieces 12 oz	Eating with family	Famished, then too full
Mon	9:00	Popcorn, cookies, 2% milk	1/2 bag 2 1 cup	TV	Bored, tired

wearing the same amount of clothing. If your weight is going up 3 weeks in a row, it is time to take a closer look at your recent food intake and physical activity.

2) Stimulus control

This is learning to identify what triggers unplanned eating and limiting exposure to these triggers. An example would be not walking down the candy aisle in the grocery store if seeing all that candy triggers you to put some in your cart. Eating in only one place, such as at the kitchen table, helps prevent unconscious eating by making you more consciously aware of when and what you are eating. Avoiding magazines or cooking shows with pictures of mouth-watering recipes helps reduce cravings.

3) Problem solving

This involves identifying problem areas, trying new solutions and evaluating their usefulness. Often, when people have a failure or "lapse" as they are changing habits, they are tempted to give up on their efforts. Instead, learning from each mistake and moving forward with this new information can help you next time you encounter a problem or high-risk situation.

4) Challenging unrealistic thoughts and beliefs

Unrealistic thoughts, beliefs and goals can undermine the best intentions and efforts. Using the example above, if a person overeats at lunch, instead of telling oneself, "I blew it, I might as well give up," it is more useful to say, "I overate at this meal, but I can still eat a healthy supper and perhaps do some extra walking tonight."

5) Rewards

Rewarding yourself as you make desired changes is very important in order to stay motivated. There can be small rewards for meeting weekly goals and larger rewards for meeting long-term goals . . . just be sure the rewards are not food! Examples of small rewards are treating yourself to a movie, book, nail polish or lipstick. Examples of rewards for meeting long-term goals are a professional massage, buying a new outfit or planning a "getaway" day or weekend.

6) Learning to manage stress

Let's face it: stress is a part of everyone's life. Without some stress, we'd be dead. The key is managing stress by learning and practicing techniques such as relaxation, deep breathing and saying no when appropriate.

7) Social support

Social support is important for support, encouragement, and accountability. Support may be informal through relatives and friends, or formal through an organized group or network.

Is a vegetarian diet a healthy way to lose weight?

In a recent five-year study of approximately 22,000 men and women in the United Kingdom, the lowest weight gain was observed in those who had changed their diet to include less animal food. A vegetarian diet can be very healthy if careful choices are made. Plant-based foods provide protein, vitamins, minerals and fiber. Nuts, seeds and oils contribute healthy fat, but it is important not to overdo these items because too much can add excess calories. If a person is eating a totally vegan diet (no animal products), it is important to obtain vitamin B-12 through fortified foods or a supplement. Careful attention should be given to consume a variety of foods containing calcium and iron. Vitamin D-fortified foods are important, as well as obtaining sufficient omega-3 fatty acids for optimum health. Suggested Web-sites to learn more about vegetarian eating are at the end of this chapter.

If I'm overweight and want to quit smoking, won't I gain weight?

Weight gain is common when quitting smoking, occurring in approximately 80 percent of those who quit. However, the weight gained from quitting smoking is less likely to result in as many negative consequences as continuing smoking, so quitting smoking is always recommended. Weight gains average from 4.5 to 7 lbs, but 13 percent of women and 10 percent of men gain more than 28 lbs. One-third of the weight gain after quitting is associated with a decrease in metabolism of approximately 100 calories daily. The remaining two-thirds of the weight gain appears to be from eating more. It is not uncommon to replace the hand-to-mouth habit with food. Also, anxiety and boredom may result in increased eating. A useful strategy would be to avoid or minimize weight gain when quitting smoking, then trying to achieve desired weight loss afterward. Short-term weight gain with quitting smoking does not rule out long-term weight control.

What questions should I ask if I am considering any weight-loss product or program?

1) Does it make weight loss promises that sound unrealistic or too good to be true (i.e., "lose 40 lbs in 30 days")? If so, it will not likely produce long-term results and may be unhealthy.
2) What is the average weight loss experienced? What is the long-term success rate?

165

3) If a diet plan is offered, is it balanced in all major food groups, or does it eliminate certain foods or food groups? Is it something that is livable, or would one tire of eating the same foods after a while?

4) Does it address eating behavior changes, exercise and other lifestyle changes for ongoing success?

5) Is it backed by qualified health professionals who are licensed in their field, such as Licensed Dietitians, or backed by reliable health organizations?

6) What is the cost or fee? Are there hidden costs which would make long-term commitment a challenge?

Are diet pills safe?

There are two broad categories of diet pills:

1) *Prescription medications* may be indicated as part of treatment for a person whose BMI (body mass index) is 30 or higher with no other risk factors or disease, or for a person whose BMI is 27-30 with other risk factors or diseases. Examples of prescription medications used for weight loss are sibutramine (Meridia), which blunts appetite, and orlistat (Xenical), which blocks the absorption of fat eaten. Any medication carries a risk of side effects, which should be discussed in detail with your physician and pharmacist before starting. What is important to remember is that all of these types of medications are meant to be used along with a healthy diet and regular exercise – they are not "magic bullets." It is common for people to regain lost weight once they discontinue these types of medications.

2) *Over-the-counter pills*. These vary in their ingredients and the claims they make for weight loss. At the very least, they are a waste of money. They may result in unhealthy and dangerous side effects and can interfere with prescription medications.

166

They are not recommended for weight loss.

When is weight-loss surgery an option?

Surgery for weight loss, called *bariatric surgery*, is considered in cases when:

1) A person's BMI is 40 or over, or
2) A person's BMI is 35-39.9 and he or she has significant health problems related to obesity, such as diabetes, high blood pressure, or sleep apnea.

Popular surgical procedures include vertical gastric banding and Roux-en-Y. The ***vertical gastric banding*** reduces stomach capacity. The ***Roux-en-Y Gastric Bypass*** reduces stomach size and bypasses part of the small intestine where calories and nutrients are absorbed. People who have Roux-en-Y Gastric bypass generally lose up to two-thirds of their excess body weight in 1-2 years following the surgery. The surgery carries significant risks. Lifelong nutritional supplementation is necessary to avoid deficiency diseases, and lifestyle changes are necessary to maintain weight loss. A multidisciplinary bariatric program – offering a team of experts including the physician, nurse, dietitian, pharmacist, psychologist and physical and recreational therapists – can meet the needs of the whole person as changes after surgery affect every facet of a person's life.

Where can I get help with my weight?

There is help available from many sources. Local hospitals and clinics, as well as some fitness centers have licensed dietitians and physical therapists that are available for individual consultation, and group programs may be available. Many employers now offer wellness programs to their employees. Some grocery stores have licensed dietitians on staff.

167

Internet resources are plentiful, but be sure to check the reliability of the site. Some suggested sites include:

American Dietetic Association
hppt://www.eatright.org

Dietary Guidelines for Americans 2005
http://www.mypyramid.gov

National Heart, Lung and Blood Institute
http://www.nhlbi.nih.gov/health/public/heart/obesity/lose_wt/index.htm

Partnership for Healthy Weight Management
http://www.consumer.gov/weightloss

Physician's Committee for Responsible Medicine (vegetarian)
http://www.pcrm.org

Shape Up America!
http://www.shapeup.org

Vegetarian Resource Group
http://www.vrg.org

Weight Control Information Network
http://www.niddk.nih.gov/health/nutrit/nutrit.htm

Remember that weight management is a life-long journey. Focus on progress, not perfection!

Chapter 13

Stay Active: The Importance of Exercise as we Age
Karen Doy, MS

Is it safe for me to start an exercise program?

Consider discussing your decision with your physician before participating in a moderate or vigorous exercise program. Moderate exercise is the amount of activity that feels about the same as walking up a flight of stairs. Also, consult your physician before starting your program if you have:

- Shortness of breath and/or fatigue at rest or with moderate activity
- Loss of balance due to dizziness or loss of consciousness
- Swelling in the ankles (or if you are on medication to reduce swelling)
- Irregular heart beat (or if you are on medication for your heart)
- Discomfort in the back of your legs that increases with walking
- Discomfort in the chest, neck, jaw, arms or other areas that increases with activity
- A known heart murmur
- Bone or joint problems that could be made worse by a change in physical activity
- Any cardiovascular risk factors (smoke, high blood pressure, high cholesterol, diabetes, overweight)
- Concerns about the safety of an exercise or activity
- Any other reason that would require you to exercise with medical supervision (for example: recent heart attack, pulmonary disease, or severe arthritis)

The consultation with your physician will help you to optimize the results of your exercise program. Improvements in endurance and intensity may be seen at any age. Exercise has the potential to greatly increase the demands upon your cardiovascular system, muscles and joints, so be safe by checking first!

What other safety measures should I take?

Think about the type of exercise you plan to do. Then take a look at the area where you plan to do that activity. Consider:

- Are there throw rugs in the way?
- Are there lamp cords that need to be moved?
- Does a path need to be cleared?
- Do I have the proper footwear?
- Do I need a cane or walker for improved balance?
- Do I need a helmet or padding?
- Are my clothes comfortable and flexible enough for the activity?
- Would I be safer exercising with someone?

Senior exercisers are more susceptible to heat injury because the elderly have a decreased ability to regulate temperature and feel thirst. Medications can make this situation worse. Drink plenty of fluids. A good rule of thumb is to consume a cup of water every 20 minutes of activity starting ½-hour before exercise.

Avoid exercise if you are running a temperature or are otherwise ill.

Exercise should feel very light to somewhat hard. If the activity feels very hard, reduce the intensity.

Particularly when just getting started, keep the activity simple and comfortable. Then, as you gain confidence, add new activities to keep exercise enjoyable and free from monotony. Activity does not have to be difficult to produce results.

You only need to be consistent in your efforts and strive to achieve steady, safe progress.

Why Should I Become More Active?

If you want to improve your health – ***think exercise!***
Physical activity promotes independence. In fact, exercise is essential in helping you to remain self-sufficient as you age. The most common reason for admission into a nursing home is the inability to get out of a chair by oneself. The American Heart Association states that every year, 12 percent of total deaths in the United States are attributed to a lack of regular physical exercise.

Some health benefits of exercise include:
- Enhanced weight control
- Better sleep
- The feeling of more energy
- Relief from depression
- Reduced stress
- Improved memory and concentration
- Better ability to fight off colds and other illnesses
- Arthritis relief
- Less risk of osteoporosis with weight-bearing activity
- Stronger muscles for better balance
- Better control over blood sugar, cholesterol and blood pressure, leading to a decreased risk of heart disease
- Less risk of colon cancer

Exercise improves the quality of life, making life more rewarding. Through exercise we are able to achieve efficiently-working muscles, allowing the joints to work more effectively with less pain and fatigue, even if the joint has some arthritis or wear and tear. This translates into being able to carry your grocery bag into the house and climb the stairs more easily.

171

More muscle means less weight gain, since muscle burns more calories than fat. Control of obesity decreases the work of the heart and improves blood sugar and cholesterol and blood pressure levels.

Think of the alternatives:
- Less muscle mass means less strength, slower movements, less coordination, poorer balance, less stamina, longer recovery time, more stiffness and soreness after exercise, altered posture, altered appearance and body proportions, the need for fewer calories and diet modification.
- Less flexibility means less stride length when walking.

How much exercise is enough?
Some activity is better than no activity. Ideally, in order to attain health benefits, aim for at least 30 minutes of moderate physical activity most, and preferably, all days of the week. A brisk walk is the most common way to achieve this result. However, there are many other ways of reaching the same goal.

Once you are comfortable with the level of activity needed to attain health benefits, work on achieving cardiovascular benefits. This requires more vigorous activity for at least 30 minutes, three days per week, along with a moderate level of physical activity most days of the week. Eventually, working your way toward high-level physical activity (>2,000 calories weekly) improves your chance of a healthy life compared with individuals with lower physical activity levels.

Pattern your activities using suggestions from the activity chart.

My Exercise Program

Exercise Element	Start With . . .	Progress Toward . . .
Type: 　-To build **endurance**, do any activity that uses the large muscle groups of your body. 　-To build **strength**, resist your body, use free weights, bands or machines. 　-To increase **flexibility,** stretch without or with aids. 　-To improve **balance**, incorporate activities that stretch your steadiness throughout the exercise session.	-Walking on land or in water, stationary cycling, recumbent stepper, etc. -Get up from and sit down in a chair, resistance bands, use soup cans as weights, etc. -Gently stretching in all directions. -Stand on one leg while holding onto something sturdy.	-Activities that take more skill such as basketball, skating, running, etc. -Resisting body weight, such as wall push-ups, sit-ups, then machines with physician approval. -Use bands, partnering, yoga, Pilates, etc. -Sit or do activities on a stability ball.
Duration	Five-minute sessions up to six times per day.	For **Health** Benefits: At least 30 minutes of activity (does not need to be continuous). For **Fitness** Benefits: Continuous activity for 30 minutes or more.

Frequency	Multiple short sessions daily	For **Health** Benefits: Daily For **Fitness** Benefits: Daily lower intensity activity and higher intensity activity several days per week.
Intensity	Fairly light	For **Health** Benefits: Fairly light to somewhat hard. For **Fitness** Benefits: Fairly light to hard.

Suggestions to help you progress safely:
- Start only one new activity per day.
- Increase duration of exercise before intensity of exercise.
- Do not increase activity by more than 10 percent per week.
- Exercise at a rate that allows you to talk to others.
- If problems occur, decrease the level of activity. See a physician if problems continue.
- Avoid burnout by exercising no more than an hour at the fairly light to somewhat hard range on a daily basis.

Most importantly, *listen to your body*. **If you are in pain – STOP!** Inform your physician if your activity results in chest pain, dizziness, shortness of breath, rapid heart rate or other symptoms that last longer than a few minutes after stopping.

How do I become more active?
Whatever your current level of activity is, you have the potential to improve. Start slowly and gradually build up your activity level. Going all-out is a sure way to burn out fast.

Determine your barriers:
- Have you set aside time for exercise?
- Are you embarrassed that you are not in very good physical condition?
- Do you need help to get started?

Determine your goals:
- Increased nerve and muscle function and loosened joints (flexibility)
- Increased heart and lung function (aerobic activity)
- Enhanced muscle strength (strength training)
- Improved health (aerobic, strength and flexibility training)
- Better balance to reduce falls (balance activities)

For the greatest success, incorporate your fitness goals into your lifestyle. What are your current activities? Do you like them? If you do, you might want to do more of these activities. If not, you might want a smorgasbord of activities to choose from to reduce the monotony of a single activity. Consider:
- Joining a yoga, Tai Chi, or other flexibility class
- Walking or hiking
- Using equipment such as a stationary bicycle or stepper
- Joining an exercise class that caters to the elderly
- Using the weight machines at a local health club
- Purchasing an exercise video or book as a guide
- "Playing" with your grandchildren or neighbor kids

Never increase the frequency, timing or intensity of your workout by more than 10 percent each week.

Exercise at a level at which you can maintain a conversation (even if it is with yourself).

If you desire more detailed instruction or just need someone to help motivate you, consider joining a class, hiring a personal trainer, exercising with a friend, or joining a monitored exercise session, such as a cardiopulmonary rehabilitation maintenance program.

Think about what you are currently doing. Think about what you enjoy doing. Think about how you are going to progress week by week, month by month. Maybe you will increase the frequency or the intensity or add an activity, but don't do all three at once!

How do I stay motivated to stay active?

Remember, your most recent activity is the one from which you derive the most benefit. What you did yesterday or today counts more than what you did last week!

Tips to keep you on target:
- Exercise with a friend. You can socialize, encourage each other, and keep each other accountable to meeting your established goal(s).
- Chart your progress by keeping an exercise log.
- Schedule your workouts, as you would an important meeting.
- Keep activity a priority in your life. Strive toward 30 minutes of activity every day.
- Keep reminding yourself of your goal(s).
- Remember inactivity leads to stiffness, soreness, less flexibility.
- The activity you choose should be accessible, convenient and enjoyable.
- Most people stop an exercise program almost as soon as they get started because they work too intensely. Take the conservative approach by starting slowly and working your way toward more intense activity.

What are the essential elements of an exercise program?

The four building blocks of an exercise program are: *endurance*, *strength*, *flexibility* and *balance*. Each is important for total fitness. If you are just starting to become more active, you will want to start with one of these elements and gradually add the others. Eventually, you will be able to include all of the elements over the course of a week on a regular basis.

Where you start depends on your current level of ability. If you are able to walk, you might want to start by walking a few minutes several times a day. If slow, light walking is difficult for you, you may want to begin with some muscle-strengthening exercises, such as sitting down and getting up from every chair at your kitchen table.

Whatever activity you choose, incorporate a short warm-up period first. A warm-up involves moving the same muscles you will be using. An example would be to sit or stand while marching in place for a few minutes.

Complete your activity with a cool-down. A cool-down (the reverse of the warm-up) is when you gradually slow down the activity you were doing. This is important to keep your muscles, including your heart, working properly. You will have less of a tendency to feel dizzy or sore if you cool down slowly. Eventually, the end of a cool-down is a perfect place to add a few flexibility exercises.

As you become more proficient at exercise, you will increase the duration and decrease the frequency of activity. A good goal to work toward would be 30 minutes of fairly light to somewhat hard activity you enjoy doing most days of the week. Once you achieve this level, you might consider reaching a vigorous level of activity for 30 to 60 minutes, 3-5 days a week. Whatever you do, do not increase your time, distance, repetitions or weight by more than 10% per week.

Let's review! Eventually your exercise routine will look like this:
- Warm-up (balance)
- Workout (endurance and/or strength and balance)
  - Type: Activities that include the large muscle groups for at least 20 minutes (walking, swimming, etc.)
  - Strength-training machines, free weights, bands, etc.
  - Stability balls, etc.
- Cool-down (balance, flexibility stretches)

Why Should I Stretch?

If you have ever had a difficult time bending over to pick something up or reaching for that object just over your head, you might have benefited from being more flexible. Flexibility comes with stretching. Stretching several times a week leads to improved performance, balance and agility. It is this habitual stretching that will reduce your risk of injury with activity. Remember to:
- Stretch safely, as overzealousness can lead to injury. This means **no bouncing**!
- Stretch after physical activity when muscles are warm and ready to lengthen and less prone to an overstretching injury.
- Breathe slowly and deeply as you stretch.
- Hold the stretch for 10 to 30 seconds and repeat the stretch up to 3 times.
- Stretch all of the major muscle groups: the calf muscles, front and back thigh muscles (quadriceps and hamstrings), hip flexors, chest (pectoral) muscles,

upper back muscles, neck, shoulder, wrists, ankles.

Other benefits of stretching include:
- Improved balance
- Better posture
- Enhanced pain relief
- Improved circulation

Common types of activities are Yoga, Pilates, ballet, Tai Chi, martial arts, swimming, and stability-ball exercises.

What is aerobic or endurance exercise?

Aerobic or *endurance exercise* is any activity that uses the large muscle groups of your body for long periods of time. That means continuous activity using the legs, trunk and/or arms for at least several minutes without stopping. Building the muscles used in the activity helps to make the *cardiorespiratory system* more efficient. Examples are:
- Walking
- Running
- Stair climbing
- Dancing
- Skating
- Aquatic exercise
- Stationary cycling
- Rowing

If your goal is to also lose weight, this is the type of activity you will want to do at a fairly light to hard level for up to sixty minutes most days of the week.

Why Strength-Train?

As we age, we can lose up to one percent of our strength per year after the age of 25. Why does this happen? Because we don't use those muscles! By including strength training in your fitness plan, you will help to develop your level of fitness and prevent injury regardless of your age. ***Muscles are trainable at any age, so it is never too late to start.*** Strength training improves muscular strength, endurance, and neuromuscular function, counteracting muscle weakness and physical frailty. A measurable difference may be seen in as few as eight weeks.

Remember to:
- Strength-train a minimum of two days per week.
- Warm up the muscles first by walking, marching, etc.
- Work all of the major muscle groups (arms, legs, chest, shoulders, back and stomach)
- Never work the same muscles two days in a row.
- Include a variety of activities such as calisthenics (push-ups, sit-ups, chin-ups), barbells, weight machines, bands, Pilates and other classes.
- Incorporate daily activities such as gardening and housework.
- Breathe normally.
- Control movements; avoid explosive movements.
- Perform the exercises in a range of motion that does not elicit pain or discomfort.

Weight machines are safer for the beginner because they "position" the body. Initially use light weights and build up gradually. The weight is too heavy if you can not repeat 8 exercises in a row with good form. The weight is too light if you can lift it more than 15 times in a row with good form. An easy number to remember to try to achieve is one set of 12 repetitions for each muscle group. You may rest and repeat a set if you want, but never do more than 3 sets. The greatest amount of conditioning is accomplished in the first set.

Where should I exercise?

Anywhere! Become more active by looking for ways to include activity into your daily routine:

- Park the car farther away than usual and walk.
- Walk instead of driving the car.
- Take the stairs instead of the elevator.
- Do a variety of household chores.
- Do stomach exercises at your desk or while watching TV.
- Stand while you talk on the phone.
- Play with your kids, grandkids, neighbor kids and friends.

For more structured activity, think about your personal preferences. Where are you most likely to stick with the program?

A fitness facility offers a variety of exercise, equipment, training advice, safe activity, and a social atmosphere. However, it may be intimidating, inconvenient and expensive. Look around for a facility that caters to your needs.

Your home is private and convenient, but you may be less safe if exercising alone.

Personal trainers may be contracted to help you with your exercise at home or in a club setting.

Contact your local hospital for a list of exercise classes that fit your need. Many offer classes for special populations (elderly, cardiac, pulmonary, diabetic, arthritic, cancer and others). These classes are safe, usually offer a variety of activities with specialized educational classes, have a built-in social network, and are inexpensive.

How can I tell if I am exercising too hard?

If you are not able to talk to someone while you are exercising, you are working too hard.

Remember to breathe while you exercise. People tend to hold their breath while they are exerting against a weight, such as lifting an object. Never hold your breath. Breathe out as you lift, push or exert.

Increase your activity level by no more than 10% each week. Significant pain should not be experienced unless the amount, duration or frequency of the exercise has changed significantly. Seek medical advice if the pain starts during exercise or continues for more than a few minutes after you stop the activity.

When you exercise for health benefits (to reduce the risk for disease), the activity should feel fairly light to somewhat hard. When you exercise for fitness benefits (to enhance cardiopulmonary status), the activity should feel fairly light to hard. Reduce activity if it feels very hard.

Each time you have a change in a medication, discuss with your physician the effect that medication might have on your heart rate. Your physician or health care provider will be able to tell you what your safe exercise heart rate range is. Be sure to have the provider help you verify that you or the machines you are using are indicating your exercise heart rate correctly.

How do I stay active when I travel?

You will need to work on your resolve during times when there is a change in your routine. One such time is when you travel. Don't worry! You will find many options available to you if you look for them:

182

- Explore the area by walking instead of driving. (Be sure to walk only in safe areas.)
- Use resistance bands. They don't take up much room in the suitcase and can be used anywhere.
- Use the hotel exercise equipment or pool.
- Do sit-ups, balance and flexibility activities in your room. These require no special equipment. You might want to pack an extra-large towel to sit on.

Does my medicine affect my ability to exercise?

Any time you are given a new prescription, ask your physician how it will affect your exercise response or routine. Medications may affect your heart rate, rhythm and blood pressure responses toward activity. You may have to time your activity around taking your medication.

Your health care provider should be able to show you how to alter your activity while continuing to receive benefits from the activity and the medication.

How should I alter my exercise routine for my medical condition?

Our bodies change physiologically as we age. Exercise routines may be compensated to take into account the cardiovascular, metabolic and orthopedic problems that may occur with advanced age.

Resting and exercise heart rates and blood pressures may be higher due to deconditioning or disease. Blood sugars may be less stable. Shortness of breath may be more evident. Work with your physician to optimize these. Exercise with your physician's approval at a lower intensity until these are stabilized. Remember, the desired exercise heart rate decreases with age, so exercise until you feel the activity is fairly light to somewhat hard. Slow down if the activity feels hard.

Reaction times are slower and recovery times are longer as we age, so start slowly and gradually increase the intensity as you feel comfortable.

Flexibility decreases with age, so warm up slowly and stretch at the end of your exercise session.

If you have not been active for a while, your percent body fat may be higher than desired. Start slowly and gradually work toward expending 2000 calories per week through activity.

Bone mass decreases with advanced age, leading to osteoporosis. Concentrating on safe balance activities and using a cane or walker, if necessary, will reduce the risk of falling.

Strength may have to be increased before attempting aerobic, flexibility or balance activities. Begin building strength by sitting down in and getting up from every chair in your house.

Eliminate more intense strength-training exercises during active periods of pain or inflammation of arthritis.

Consider joining an aquatic exercise program. Water is very easy on the joints and is a safe way to increase muscle strength. Use slip-resistant water shoes to prevent the risk of falling.

Stationary cycling and sitting stepping machines are a great way to get a workout if it is difficult to walk.

You may accomplish more by initially attempting intermittent activity. For instance, if you have pain in your calves when you walk, walk for a few minutes, rest until the pain in your calves is gone, walk for a few minutes, rest, walk and rest. Continue this cycle until you have walked 30 minutes for the day.

What if I stop exercising for a while?

When returning from a layoff of more than three weeks, start at 50% or less of your previous time or intensity, and then gradually increase until you reach your previous level.

Remember: Any movement is better than no movement at all!

Good luck . . . and keep moving!

Alternative Medicine:
What You Need to Know
John W. Golden, MD

What is Alternative Medicine?

Alternative Medicine is a term that is applied to all "unconventional" therapies that are not taught in a "traditional" Medical School. Personally, I do not like this term for two reasons. First, it implies that there are two different types of medicine, and, second, it suggests that there might be a right and a wrong way to provide healthcare and that the two are incompatible.

Having said that, I prefer the term "*Complementary Medicine*," because it suggests that although there are different schools of thought, there is benefit from combining them for the betterment of the patient.

My favorite term, however, is "*Integrative Medicine*," because it says that all forms of therapy have value and that the best needs of the patient are served by a skillful blending of the best of Conventional Medicine and Complementary Therapies.

Currently, there are several training programs throughout the United States that are preparing physicians in this new and exciting specialty. Many people believe that Integrative Medicine is the "medicine of the future" because it offers a wider variety of options for the clinician, beyond the traditional paradigm of medications and surgery.

What is Integrative Medicine?

Integrative Medicine has four basic principles:

1. First, **Integrative Medicine emphasizes healing, not curing**. The conventional medical model, with its emphasis on technology, focuses on curing. Curing is the absence of disease. Healing is a concept which implies a return to holism, a sense of peace and acceptance of what is. Curing is not always possible, but healing always is. Furthermore, Integrative Medicine recognizes that the body, if given the proper conditions, possesses everything it needs to heal. Our role, as physicians, is to enhance the body's natural ability to heal.

2. Second, **Integrative Medicine treats the patient as an equal partner in the healing relationship**. I, as the physician, bring my expertise in various disease states to the relationship. Correspondingly, the patient brings his/her expertise in their own individual expression of disease. Together, we put together a unique therapeutic plan for that individual. Integrative Medicine is not one-size-fits-all medicine.

3. Third, **Integrative Medicine looks at the patient from a holistic perspective**. You see, each of us is a multidimensional person. We are physical, emotional, mental, and spiritual beings. In order to evaluate the patient fully, we have to consider not only each of these dimensions individually, but, also, how each affects the others.

4. Fourth, **Integrative Medicine views all disease as a process, not an event**. Whenever we look at a disease, we need to consider where on the continuum the disease state is. From that understanding, it is much easier to plan a treatment course.

5. Finally, within this framework, **Integrative Medicine employs the various conventional and complementary therapies in cooperation with the patient to create the unique clinical course for that patient**.

Having done a two-year Fellowship in Integrative Medicine at the University of Arizona, I have brought these skills to my practice and have found that many of my patients are already seeing a variety of Complementary providers, such as Chiropractors, Massage Therapists, Acupuncturists and Oriental Medicine practitioners. For the most part, however, there is no communication between or among the providers. The ability to understand the language and terminology of these other disciplines allows me to serve as a coordinator of care for my patients, as well as to answer some of their questions.

In order to help you understand this discipline, I will share with you some of the most common questions I am asked by patients.

What are the most common Alternative or Complementary Therapies?

There are multitudes of *Complementary and Alternative Medicine (CAM)* options available to the curious patient. Some have established themselves due to their cultural and traditional use. Others are of more recent origin, but have been researched and shown to have merit. The criterion that I use in considering a therapy is that it must have evidence of both safety and effectiveness. How I choose one or the other is based on the patient, the problem, and the goals we set together. Here is a list of how they are frequently classified:

- **Traditional or Cultural Systems**
  Ayurveda – traditional Indian Medicine
  Oriental Medicine
  Native American Medicine

- **Manual Medicine**
  Osteopathic Manipulation
  Chiropractic
  Massage Therapy

- **Lifestyle Interventions**
  Diet
  Exercise
  Nutritional Supplements

- **Mind-Body Therapies**
  Hypnosis
  Biofeedback
  Guided Imagery
  Spirituality

- **Botanical Medicine**
  Herbs

- **Energy Medicine**
  Homeopathy
  Reiki
  Healing Touch
  Acupuncture

In the interest of space, and because some of these are addressed elsewhere, I will not discuss all of these therapies but will focus on the ones I am asked about the most.

I have a friend that sees a Chiropractor. What do they do?

Chiropractic is based on the principle that health and disease are related to structure and function of the spinal column. The amount of health one experiences is proportional to the degree that the spinal column is aligned and to which there is limitation of inflammation.

According to Chiropractic philosophy, the body has an innate ability to heal itself. That ability is compromised by local injury at the spinal segmental levels. The nature of such injury may be traumatic, degenerative, or compressive. It has also been described in stress or other emotional circumstances. The injury, in turn, creates segmental derangement, or *subluxation*, a term used to define the disruption at the local spinal level. A cascade of inflammation ensues which causes swelling, limitation of movement, and spinal nerve irritation. As the problem becomes more chronic, the derangement may affect the tissues innervated by the spinal nerve that originates at that segment. This, in turn, explains the persistence of symptoms that occurs even after the acute inflammation has diminished.

Chiropractic therapy consists of a large variety of techniques, using specialized tables and instruments, and featuring much individualization between practitioners. *Spinal Manipulative Therapy* is the term used to encompass all types of techniques used by Chiropractors. *Mobilization* is a slow, passive movement within the normal range of motion. *Manipulation*, or adjustment, as it is commonly called, is a mechanical movement of a joint in a particular range and direction, usually by hand, that often produces the "pop" that patients experience. Both mobilization and manipulation are used to realign segmental derangement and, thus, to facilitate joint motion.

191

Medical referrals to Chiropractors have been limited in the past because of a perception that it was an unscientific form of therapy. However, a large body of literature has demonstrated the benefits of chiropractic treatment, especially in low-back pain, neck pain and headaches. More and more, the gap between the two disciplines is shrinking and there is the beginning of a collegial relationship.

Does Acupuncture work?

Acupuncture is only one part of a larger healing system, *Oriental Medicine*, which also includes *diet therapy, herbal therapy, exercise techniques (Tai Chi and Qi Gong), medical massage (Tui Na)*, and *meditation*. Acupuncture uses a series of precisely placed needles into defined energy channels, called *Meridians*. There are 14 principal meridians with 361 documented basic acupuncture points on the surface of the body, each with its own name and function.

The basis of Acupuncture is that *life force energy*, *Qi (pronounced CHI)*, circulates throughout the body in Meridians. These meridians, in turn, interact with internal organs deep inside the body. Health or disease is defined by whether the meridians are open or blocked and whether Qi is stagnant, deficient, or in excess. Qi is defined as different from blood, lymph, or other bodily fluids defined in Western medicine. Currently, there are no techniques in Western Medicine to measure this energy.

Acupuncture has been practiced in Asia for thousands of years. It came to the West in the 1970s due to a reporter's experience. While traveling with President Nixon in China, the reporter developed appendicitis and had acupuncture for pain relief. He was so dazzled by his experience that he reported it on the front page of **The Washington Post**, and America's fascination with Acupuncture was born.

There are multiple schools of Acupuncture, some of which only focus on one part of the body, like the ear or hand. In addition, there are different ways to stimulate the acupuncture points, including *needles, electric current, acupressure (rubbing or pressing on the point)*, *pellets* or *laser*.

Although in Chinese Medicine there are countless conditions treated with Acupuncture, the World Health Organization describes over 40 conditions in which Acupuncture's usefulness has been supported by scientific evidence. These include pain syndromes, arthritis, and a variety of other conditions. Some studies have shown the pain-relieving properties of acupuncture in conditions like arthritis surpass the pain-relieving effects of some pain medications.

Many people are intimidated by the concept of having needles placed in their body. I can assure you from personal experience that the needles are so fine that they go in without any discomfort. If you have a painful condition, I would recommend you give acupuncture a try.

What are the benefits of Massage Therapy?

Massage therapy is one of the oldest forms of therapy known to man. As long as we have been interactive, there has been healing attached to the placement of hands and the massaging of muscles. Some of the oldest recorded medical writings have included narratives on the healing power of massage.

Massage Therapy heals by assessing the soft tissues and, using scientifically based techniques of local movement and pressure, thus normalizing them. The techniques are useful for all the body systems, especially the musculoskeletal, circulatory, lymphatic, and nervous system. Through massage, the muscles are relaxed, toxins contained in the muscles are mobilized, and circulation and lymphatic

193

drainage of those toxins is accomplished.

As mentioned, touch is the most therapeutic part of massage. However, the art of massage is the ways in which that touch is applied. Sensitive touch allows the detection of a great deal of information, including areas of inflammation, muscle tension, and stress. Touch also conveys caring, which is an essential ingredient of the healing process.

There are many different methods of massage which differ in the placement of the hands and the degree of pressure applied. Over centuries, the science of massage therapy has described the right ways to massage but also has demonstrated that there are wrong or toxic methods of massage.

There are over 100 forms of Massage Therapy, and about 75% are less than 20 years old. As technology evolves and our ability to measure the outcomes of new techniques increases, newer styles are developing all the time. In general, Massage Therapy schools arise from one of five categories:

Traditional European: Probably the best known form of Massage Therapy, this is based on conventional concepts of Anatomy and Physiology, incorporating five basic techniques: ***Effleurage (gliding strokes), Petrissage (kneading), Friction (rubbing), Tapotement (percussion)***, and ***Vibration***. An example would be Swedish massage.

Contemporary Western: Based on more modern understandings of human functioning, and using a wide variety of manipulative techniques, including mind/body work, as well. Examples include ***Neuromuscular Massage, Manual Lymph Drainage, Sports massage***, and ***Myofascial release***.

194

Structural, Functional, and Movement Integration:
Using gravity and other positional relationships to correct inappropriate patterns of movement, as well as balancing the nervous system through new patterns of movement. An example would be Rolfing.

Oriental: Based on Traditional Oriental Medical principles of treating the energetic flow within the body. The trained use of pressure and manipulation along the energy channels allows for the balancing of energy flow and healing. Examples include *Shiatsu, Acupressure*, and *Tui Na*.

Energetics: Based on the belief that the body consists of and is surrounded by an energetic field and that disruptions or imbalances in this field can affect health. The practitioner uses touch in and through this energetic field to balance and correct energy derangements. Examples include *Therapeutic Touch, Healing Touch*, and *Reiki*.

Massage Therapy has been studied and found to be safe in all age groups, from the prenatal period through old age. Many conditions have been shown to be helped by this discipline. Some conditions in which to avoid Massage, however, include active infection or acute inflammation where the massage might enhance spread. Cancer is a controversial area for massage because of the possibility of enhancing lymphatic spread of tumor cells. There is a great deal of discussion about whether that is a theoretical or distinct possibility. Frankly, I have mixed feelings about the controversy. I respect the possibility of tumor spread, but also value the therapeutic aspects of touch. As a result, I currently recommend only gentle superficial massage, if at all, for areas surrounding the tumor, and prefer a more energetic massage such as Reiki or Healing Touch in these patients.

One other point that needs to be made involves the confusion between massage parlors and Massage Therapy. Many people have heard about this more sordid and sensual aspect of massage parlors and equate that with Massage Therapy. Nothing could be farther from the truth. Again, I want to emphasize that Massage Therapy is a scientifically-based healing discipline, and a Certified Massage Therapist is a valuable member of the healing team.

My neighbor has a child with recurrent ear infections and has used Homeopathy to help. Is there anything to that?

Homeopathy is a practical system of healing developed by Samuel Hahnemann in the early 1800s after years of personal research. It is based on the presumption that each individual possesses a self-healing ability, or vital force. Homeopathy works by activating this intrinsic ability. The self-healing ability allows the individual to return to balance, but also creates limitations. Homeopathy is only able to work within the limits of the individual's self-healing ability.

While working as a translator of medical texts in 1790, Hahnemann was intrigued with a theory about the use of cinchona bark as a treatment of malaria. To test his theory, he took cinchona bark himself and recorded his symptoms. To his amazement, he developed a group of symptoms very similar to malaria. He remembered how Hippocrates, the father of modern medicine, had described "The Law of Similars" in which he proposed that drugs that produce symptoms in healthy people will treat similar symptoms in sick people. Hahnemann went on to test, or "prove," other substances, the results of which he carefully chronicled and later published.

From his experiments, Hahnemann created a system of

healing based on several laws:

The Law of Similars: In order for the "drug" to act homeopathically, the "proved" symptoms of the remedy must be exactly matched to the symptoms of the patient. This includes not only the general physical symptoms, but also the specifics, like location, mitigating factors, and other areas of the body involved. In addition, mental, emotional and any other concomitant symptoms must be included in the description of the process. Because of the specificity of remedy, the initial interview, or constitutional case-taking, by a homeopathic practitioner often takes 1 to 2 hours. Hahnemann carefully cataloged his individual remedies into a large volume called the *Homeopathic Pharmocopeia* which, at last printing, includes over 1000 substances. Classical Homeopathy uses substances individually. Although combination remedies are available today, Hahnemann always emphasized using one remedy at a time and discouraged the use of combination remedies.

Single Dose: Hahnemann taught that one dose would stimulate the body and create a change. It was important for the practitioner to be patient and observant, but most of all resist the temptation to repeat the treatment too soon. To do so could inactivate or interfere with the healing response.

Minimum dose: Another of the basic laws states that the lowest possible dose should be used to stimulate the healing response. Too high a dose or additional doses would render the remedy ineffective.

The Laws of Cure: This basic tenet holds that removal of symptoms is not enough; the objective of treatment is cure. In addition, disease moves in a particular direction as it progresses, and correspondingly, moves in the opposite direction as it is cured. It moves from the more vital organs

197

to the less vital organs, from within to without, from above to below, and in the reverse order of appearance. This gives the practitioner markers to observe the effectiveness of the treatment.

The Law of Dilution and Succussion: This is one of the most difficult laws for the conventional practitioner to understand. Hahnemann was concerned that some of the substances used were poisonous, and tried to find the minimal dose required to be effective. He noted that diluted remedies not only produced fewer side effects, but they also maintained their medicinal properties. Hahnemann also discovered that by *succussing* (vigorously shaking or striking the dissolved remedy), an increase in healing power occurred. The more the medication is diluted and succussed, the stronger the remedy becomes. There are three categories of homeopathic potencies: X potencies (diluted 1 part per 10), C potencies (diluted 1 part per 100), and M (diluted 1 part per 1000). This is where the sticking point is for many conventional practitioners. Much of the controversy relates to how such a diluted concentration can have an effect. Much of the result has been ascribed by conventional practitioners to the *Placebo effect*, because with enough dilutions, there is literally none of the initial substance in the solution.

In truth, we do not know how Homeopathy works. Supporters attribute the mechanism of action to "Smart Water." According to this belief, every substance, when dissolved in a solvent, leaves a unique energetic imprint of itself within the solvent. The repetitive dilution and succussion enhances this vibrational imprint and strengthens its potency.

Whatever the mechanism, there have been double-blinded studies which attest to the effectiveness of Homeopathy in various conditions. Homeopathy is safe, with no known side effects if the proper remedy is used. The common reasons that someone would choose Homeopathy include disliking conventional "drugs," wanting a "safer" remedy, looking for a less costly alternative, wanting a more holistic approach, and a provider who spends more time. Assuming that the person has a strong enough vital force, Homeopathy may offer an effective alternative. There are nonclassical homeopathic preparations available at your local health food store or pharmacy. Assuming that a person has an acute, self-limited disease, an introductory book on Homeopathy or a nonclassical combination product may be adequate. However, anyone with a chronic disease is advised to seek care from a qualified professional.

Is Herbal Medicine safe?

Herbal Medicine is defined by the European Union as "medicinal products containing as active ingredients exclusively plant products and/or vegetable matter." In reality, herbal medicine is the oldest form of medicine on the planet. As long as humans have inhabited this planet, they have lived surrounded by plant life. Herbal remedies have developed through experimentation, cultural and family traditions, and anecdotal reports. As civilizations developed, there were designated "keepers" of the secrets – Medicine Men and Women who were charged to investigate and pass on these healing secrets to subsequent generations. In fact, Herbal remedies are the foundation of many of the cultural and traditional Medical systems, such as Oriental, Indian, and Native American healing traditions. According to the World Health Organization, 80% of the world's population has plant based therapies medicine as part of its "conventional "Medicine." What we consider "conventional Medicine" is Alternative Medicine for that large population!

At the beginning of the 20th Century, physicians commonly used herbal remedies as their major form of treatment. Gradually, however, as the use of pharmaceutical preparations became more prominent, the use of herbs became increasingly scarce. This has not been the case in Western Europe, where approximately 30-40% of people use herbs as their mainstay therapy. In fact, the governments of France and Germany, in particular, have devoted great resources to the investigation and validation of herbal preparations as part of the professional arsenal of their physicians.

In this country, there has been resurgence in the interest in herbal remedies over the last twenty years. This interest has been fueled by several factors:

1. First, there is a belief that "Natural" is safer than pharmaceutical. While this is mostly true, natural remedies still should be used with discretion, and should always be disclosed to your personal healthcare provider.

2. Second, herbs are cheaper than medications. This is for the most part true, even when prescription co-pays and discounts are included. As the cost of health care continues to rise, people are looking for alternatives to control costs.

3. Third, there is an ever-increasing wealth of information available to the consumer on the Internet promoting the value of herbs over medicines. The problem comes in filtering out the good from the bad information that is available.

4. Fourth, there is a distrust in pharmaceuticals that has been born out of the increasing "direct to consumer" advertising combined with the high profile withdrawal of medications, such as Vioxx. In other words,

people are more familiar with the new medications that are prominently advertised. When some of those same medications get withdrawn, amidst the loud background of class action suits, people are becoming more suspicious of the development and approval of prescription medications.

In some of the large studies that have measured consumer preference, there have been significant increases in the public's favorable attitude and use of herbal remedies. This trend, however, has not been accompanied by the same level of interest on the part of conventional physicians. In truth, there has been a backlash of articles questioning the validity of remedies that have been used for many generations.

The pharmaceutical industry has little interest in researching plants as remedies because they cannot be patented. Therefore, the information gained cannot be used only by that company. Instead, they have focused on isolating active constituents, purifying them and acquiring a patent for them. According to several sources, as many as 40% of our known pharmaceuticals have been developed in this way.

Herbal medicines, or *phytomedicines*, are made from plant materials, for the majority of which the active ingredient is unknown. They may contain a single biologically active compound, or their effect may be due to a complex mixture of compounds whose combined effects produce the end result. The amount of active constituents may vary due to a host of factors, including soil type, sun exposure, rain amounts, timing of collection, temperature, maturity of the plant, associated surrounding plant life, and storage conditions. It is felt that the level of constituent chemicals is derived by these factors because they provide the plant with an advantage against other plants, as well as natural conditions like insects, sunlight, drought, etc. In general, the

201

active constituents are present in lower concentrations than purified, single ingredient pharmaceuticals. This is one of the factors that contribute to lower risks than a single purified compound.

Another is the fact that many of the compounds work to balance the effect of another compound in the same plant. For instance, among the many helpful ingredients in green tea is *caffeine*. As we all know, caffeine is a biologically active stimulant. Also present, however, is an amino acid, *L-theanine*, which has a calming but non-sedating effect which balances the stimulant side effect of the caffeine.

Herbal medicines are available in many forms and are made from whole plants, plant parts, or extracts or concentrates of active plant compounds. They are available as fresh plants, as well as in solid or liquid forms. Fresh plants are typically prepared as an infusion, in which boiling water is poured over the plant and allowed to steep, as in a tea. A decoction is a little different in that the plant is boiled in water and then the excess remaining material is strained off, leaving the active compounds in the liquid. Other liquid forms include medicinal oils, medicinal spirits, plant juices, syrups and tinctures, and glycerites. Solid forms are available as powders – either whole plant or extracts, and concentrates, and can be administered as granules, coated or uncoated tablets, capsules, or lozenges.

In addition, many herbal products are standardized, meaning they contain a percentage of an ingredient used either as a reference marker of quality or as a measure of an active ingredient. They may be purchased either as a single ingredient product or as a combination product, where two or more herbs are combined for additive or synergistic effect.

Table 1: Top-Selling Herbal Dietary Supplements in the Food, Drug, and Mass Market Retail Channels in 2004 (for 52-weeks ending January 2, 2005)*

Rank/Herb	Dollar Sales
1. Garlic	$27,013,420
2. Echinacea	$23,782,640
3. Saw Palmetto	$20,334,030
4. Ginkgo	$19,334,010
5. Soy	$17,419,530
6. Cranberry	$13,445,670
7. Ginseng [†]	$12,165,220
8. Black Cohosh	$11,984,960
9. St. John's wort	$9,087,829
10. Milk thistle	$7,775,529
11. Evening primrose	$6,088,103
12. Valerian	$3,449,297
13. Green tea	$2,794,783
14. Bilberry	$2,341,301
15. Grape seed	$2,330,281
16. Horny goat weed	$2,203,555
17. Yohimbe	$1,835,313
18. Horse Chestnut	$1,564,550
19. Eleuthero	$992,286
20. Ginger	$814,789
Multi-Herbs [‡]	$52,049,290
All other herbs	$11,841,120
Total Herb Supplements	$257,514,900

* Data courtesy <u>Information Resources, Inc.</u>, Chicago, IL. All data are based on sales in FDM channel for 52-week period ending Jan. 2, 2005. Data do not include sales from Wal-Mart stores, or sales from other market channels: health and natural food stores, mail order, MLM companies, health professionals, warehouse buying clubs, and convenience stores.

† Presumably includes Asian ginseng (Panax ginseng) and American ginseng (P. quinquefolius)

‡ Multi-herbs refers to combination formulations containing more than one herb.

A recent survey by Information Resources, Inc., examined herbal sales in 2004. Table 1 is the ranking of the 20 top-selling herbs and the dollars spent.

There is a misconception amongst the consuming public that because herbal remedies are "natural" they are also harmless. And while it is true that there are fewer adverse reaction reports filed for herbals than pharmaceuticals, it would be erroneous to believe that they are free of side effects. Moreover, because their ingredients are chemicals, they are processed and removed from the body using the same metabolic pathways as medications. Therefore, there is the potential for drug-herb interactions, which could enhance side effects of the herb, the medication, or both. This point is especially important because a recent study suggested that as many as 60% of patients taking herbal therapies do not report them to their physician because they believe them to be of no concern.

There are several areas of concern related to the use of herbal medicine:

1. First, under current FDA guidelines, herbs fall outside the regulatory guidelines of the FDA. Therefore, there is no guarantee of the purity, or potency of the product. In addition, because herbs are derived from plants, differences in growing conditions can lead to variability in the potency of the same herb between batches from the same manufacturer.

2. Second, the potency of the product is usually related to the part of the plant used, and some manufacturers do not include this important point on the labeling. Product mislabeling, adulterations, and misidentification have occurred. Furthermore, there is confusion between the use of the whole plant or standardized extract of the herb. In general, a "standardized extract" will contain a

measured amount of an active ingredient which has been shown to correlate to activity.

3. Third, the use of herbs in pregnancy, breastfeeding, in children, and in serious medical conditions should only be used under the direction of a trained professional, because of the potential for harmful side effects. In any case, any herbal medicine should be stopped if any side effects should occur.

Some of my favorite herbal remedies include Saw Palmetto for symptoms of enlarged prostate in men; Black Cohosh for post-menopausal symptoms in women; Echinacea for viral infections; St. John's Wort for mild to moderate depression; Ginger for nausea, motion sickness, and its anti-inflammatory effect; and Valerian root for insomnia. None of these should be used without some personal research into side effects and interactions. In addition, if you are taking medications, check with your physician for any interactions.

A listing of the most common herbal remedies and their indications can be found at the website of the ***American Botanical Council***, www.herbalgram.org. Other resources include "The Healing Power of Herbs" and "The Encyclopedia of Natural Medicine," by Michael Murray, N.D.

Should I be taking Supplements? And, if so, which ones?

Supplements are just that, a supplement, or a part of a healthy lifestyle. Contrary to the claims of some, they, by themselves are not the answer to health problems. I will go so far as to say that a person will be healthier following a healthy lifestyle without supplements than taking supplements and following an unhealthy lifestyle. Having said that, I still recommend supplements to complement the rest of a person's health plan, but I think that any supplement plan should be goal-directed. I have had people come into my office literally with two shopping bags full of supplements. When I ask them why they take them, the response is usually something like, "I read about them in a magazine," or, "I saw it on TV." Typically, most people have no recollection why they are taking most of the products. In addition, when thinking about supplements, you need to think in terms of maintenance or therapeutic reasons. In other words, are you taking the supplement for day-to-day maintenance of function, or are you taking the supplement to accomplish some therapeutic endpoint?

With that prelude, here is the list of the basic supplements I recommend:

1. First, and foremost, as a maintenance supplement, I recommend a ***comprehensive multivitamin and mineral preparation***. For this purpose, I regularly discourage the typical one-tablet-a-day multi, unless, as I tell my patients, it's as big as a golf ball. The reason for this is that most one-tablet-a-day multivitamins are designed to be maintenance products. In other words, they assume that you are getting the vast majority of your nutrients from your diet; that your activity and stress levels are consistent; and that you have no pre-existing deficiencies of nutrients. As you can imagine, this description applies to very few individuals. For the majority, there is inconsistency in diet, activity, stress, and, in a large percentage of people, preexisting nutritional deficiencies. In my mind, it is better to take more nutrients than you body needs and let it decide what is important than to find your body wanting for more than is delivered.

2. Second, I recommend ***fish oil***. We live in a society that encourages inflammation. The typical American diet is rich in a type of polyunsaturated fat called Omega-

6, which has pro-inflammatory effect, thickens the blood, and constricts blood vessels. While this type of reaction might be important in certain situations, such as infection, or bleeding, for most of us it increases our risk of inflammation. By contrast, there is another type of polyunsaturated fat called Omega-3, which has the exact opposite effect: anti-inflammatory, thins blood, and dilates blood vessels. This type of effect is important in preventing inflammation. Both types of fat are essential for human health but must exist in balance. Medical historians tell us that in ancient times, when our ancestors were hunter/gatherers, these types of fats existed in a ratio of 1:1 to 4:1 (omega-6:omega-3). In the typical American diet, these ratios range from 20:1 to as much as 40:1. The primary sources of omega-6 are corn, soy, canola, safflower and sunflower oil; these oils are overabundant in the typical diet, which explains our excess omega-6 levels. Fish Oil is a natural, highly potent source of omega-3 oils. Good sources of omega-3 also include cold water fish — such as salmon, mackerel, tuna, sardines — as well as walnuts and flaxseed oil, among others.

The choice between fish and fish oil is currently controversial. Many critics suggest avoiding fish because of the potential of contamination from heavy metals and environmental toxins. Pond-raised fish would seem to be safer, but in actuality are not, due to feedings that are high in the same contaminants. Another disadvantage is that pond-raised fish are not exposed to the cold temperature that occur at the depths where these fish typically live, and therefore contain lower levels of the essential fats. Although I recommend fish, I usually advise patients to question sellers about the origin of the fish.

3. Another supplement that may need to be supplemented is ***Calcium with Vitamin D*** for osteoporosis. Multiple

factors in our society conspire to create calcium deficiencies. Much of our diet, rather than helping in this regard, actually conspires against us. Something as common as soda pop, which is high in phosphoric acid, actually may leech the calcium out of our bones. In addition, a high-fat diet and sedentary lifestyle also contributes to low calcium levels which must be corrected by our bones contributing calcium. Vitamin D, essential for calcium absorption, is processed in our skin, and requires sunlight to activate the process. The increased fear of skin cancers, plus the increased use of sunscreens, which inhibit this process, contribute to low vitamin D levels and thus increases the risk of osteoporosis.

4. ***Magnesium*** is another important mineral to supplement. Studies have shown that as many as 86% of our elderly population is deficient in magnesium. Magnesium is an important regulator of muscle activity in the body. Deficiency is associated with increased muscle spasms and cramping. More importantly, because the heart is a muscle, low levels of magnesium may contribute to irregularities of heart rhythm.

5. Another maintenance supplement that has generated a lot of controversy is the class of ***Antioxidants***. This is a group of supplements which includes ***Vitamins A, C, E, and the mineral Selenium***. This group has its benefits from the neutralization of a group of chemicals called Free Radicals. Free Radicals are unstable compounds that arise through a variety of causes, including diet, sunlight, aging, vigorous aerobic exercise, as well as others. The theory says that these chemicals are unstable and pull electrons from cells and other chemicals causing cellular injury. Most people agree with this mechanism. Where the controversy ensues is how much antioxidant material do we need?

There have been two opposing views. The first has said that because we live in a society where free radicals are everywhere, we should be taking large doses of antioxidants to protect ourselves from cellular damage. The other, more recent viewpoint, is that free radicals are a double-edged sword. They not only can do the damage that the other school describes, but they are also part of our own defense mechanisms against things like various infections and cancer. According to this view, it is possible to take too many antioxidants, and thus weaken our own defenses.

As you can imagine, this creates a great deal of confusion, especially since there have been some studies suggesting that the use of single antioxidants, i.e., Vitamin C or Betacarotene alone have increased the risk of cancers. My recommendations are that you never take Antioxidants in isolation; always take a blend. In fact, some antioxidants are members of families which together provide more effect. Examples include *mixed carotenoids* instead of Beta Carotene, and *mixed tocopherols* instead of Vitamin E. In addition, at this time, I usually counsel against the use of mega-doses of Antioxidants because of the reasons mentioned above; but I recommend more than the Daily Value (DV), which is the amount needed to prevent deficiency. In your particular situation, I recommend that you check with a knowledgeable health care provider who is familiar with your personal health history.

6. *Other supplements are used based on the person's therapeutic goals.* There are a lot of supplements, but the buyer needs to beware that there are a lot of unscrupulous people touting supplements for which there is little scientific background. Some of my favorite supplements include *Glucosamine sulfate* for arthritis;

209

Chromium for diabetes; **Coenzyme Q10** for heart issues and statin-related muscle pain; and **Melatonin** for sleep problems. I also like **Calcium d-glucarate** for enhancing detoxification and **muramyl peptides** for keeping our immune systems alert.

I go to the health food store and there literally are walls of supplements. How do I choose?

If you are considering using dietary supplements, your best weapon is education. There are a lot of supplements but not all of them are good. First, you need to be clear about what you want to accomplish. Second, you need to understand the risks and benefits of the supplements and how they fit in your particular health scenario. Third, you should consult with your health provider. Gather as much information as possible about your choice, and ask for an open discussion.

Unfortunately, many health providers are not familiar with dietary supplements, so the discussion may not go as planned. If your question is met with disdain or you are given an answer such as, "It's just expensive urine," you are probably dealing with someone unwilling to explore these options as a therapeutic partner. I would advise you to look elsewhere. All decisions should be made between you and a sympathetic care provider.

Having said that, there are several indicators of quality. First, look for the use of pharmaceutical grade ingredients. There are three grades of nutritional ingredients: food, veterinary, and pharmaceutical. Think of them as good, better, and best. They refer to the quality and purity of the ingredients used. Correspondingly, as the quality increases, so does the cost. The best value is with pharmaceutical-grade ingredients. Second, the government has established regulations called **Good Manufacturing Processes (GMP)**, which are

210

tandards for the manufacturing of dietary supplements. n general, they fall about midway between the standards or food manufacturing and the stringent FDA standards or pharmaceuticals. GMP on the label is one indicator of quality.

Third, the US Pharmacopeia (USP) is a well-known organization dedicated to producing quality control standards or the strength, quality, and purity of pharmaceuticals. n 1997, the USP began publishing standards for dietary supplements. These standards focus on the strength, quality, purity, packaging and labeling of dietary supplements and are updated yearly. USP on the label is another good indicator of quality.

Last, you should look for a well-known and reputable company. Larger companies have a national reputation o uphold and are more likely to follow high-quality manufacturing practices. In addition, don't buy the least expensive supplements. Usually this means a lower-quality ingredient or manufacturing. Remember, cheaper is not better!

Be an educated consumer! Here are more guidelines to consider when choosing supplements:

1. **Try to avoid self-diagnosis.** This could lead you into the trap of trying everything you read about or see on TV.

2. **Avoid the "quick fix"** often promised on TV infomercials; always check with your physician before you take out your credit card.

3. Also, remember: **if something sounds too good to be true, it probably is.** Always look for more information.

4. **Remember that safety is your first concern.** Before

taking any supplements, look into possible interactions with other supplements or medications you may be taking. Do not substitute a supplement for a medication without checking with your doctor first. And, it doesn't hurt to say it again: "Natural" doesn't always mean safe or free of side effects.

There are a lot of quality supplements with tremendous health benefits out there. Hopefully, these guidelines will help you not feel so intimidated when you walk into your local retailer.

What is Reiki?

Reiki [pronounced RAY-kee] is an easy-to-learn, natural, hands-on system of healing developed by Mikao Usui, a Physician and devout Zen Buddhist. After originating in Japan, Reiki teachings have been successively passed down from teacher to student for over one hundred years, and today, practitioners can be found all over the globe. It is a simple system, which once learned can be practiced on yourself, as well on others. In addition, with advanced training, you can learn to send Reiki to others anywhere in the world.

Ki is the Japanese term for the energy that flows through all things. Reiki is the term used for the healing modality that accesses and transmits this universal energy. This universal energy is transmitted through the trained practitioner and can be used for healing. The Reiki practitioner acquires his or her ability to control the healing energy through a series of trainings and attunements, which, in effect, turn on the ability to use the Reiki energy.

Although Reiki is a spiritual healing system, it is independent and unrelated to any religious system, and is definitely not a religious doctrine on its own. Nevertheless, Reiki cknowledges the source of all healing as originating from higher power. Therefore, it is important to recognize the esponsibility that accompanies being a Reiki practitioner. s mentioned, Reiki is a holistic system that complements any other healing disciplines. Its focus is on relaxation and elieving suffering. It only requires the placement of hands n the recipient by the practitioner. The healing energy flows asily and effortlessly. In fact, the recipient does not have to elieve in Reiki to gain benefit! It should also be noted that eiki energy is intelligent energy – that is, it is provided to ie recipient to be used for the highest good. Reiki can never e used for evil purposes, because that would be incongruent ith the nature of the universal energy.

eiki practitioners fall into three levels:

. ***Reiki First Degree*** is the first level of Reiki training. In this attunement, the student is initiated and aligned with the Universal Energy. The student will often feel the energy pass through him, and may describe it as warmth, tingling, or a mild vibration.

. ***Reiki Second Degree*** is the next level. Usually before attaining this level, the First Degree Reiki practitioner must practice and refine the skills that were acquired for a period of time and must self-treat with Reiki on a daily basis. The Second Degree attunements strengthen the flow of Reiki and allow the practitioner to perform Reiki treatments from a distance. In addition, the practitioner learns three symbols which help to focus the energy for the healing purposes. The use of these symbols, combined with the strengthening of the flow of energy, allows the Second Degree practitioner to heal from a distance by visualizing the recipient and directing the energy to them.

. ***Reiki Third Degree*** is considered the Master level. With increasing knowledge and strengthening of the Reiki practitioner comes more responsibility. At this level, the student has the opportunity for advanced training to rise to the level of teacher. With that comes the responsibility of passing on the Reiki lineage. There are additional symbols and attunements that accompany this level.

Reiki training is nothing more than a diploma unless there is intent for self development on the part of the student. Reiki is a healing art, but more than that, it is a path of awakening. The student is taught methods of self purification that allow them to pursue a life of meaning. When Dr. Usui developed Reiki, he had five principles he required his students to follow. Those principles, upon which Reiki is established, are still taught today. They are:

- *Just for today, do not anger.*
- *Just for today, do not worry.*
- *Honor your parents, teachers, and elders.*
- *Earn your living honestly.*
- *Show gratitude to every living thing.*

As you can see, these are principles which demand self-awareness and self-discovery. It is through the pursuit of these principles that the Reiki practitioner achieves enlightenment and fulfillment.

A typical Reiki session may last up to an hour. During it, the recipient stays dressed. Often, the lights are dimmed and soft music is played in the background. Prior to starting, the practitioner will discuss with the recipient the goals and expectations of the session. When the treatment starts, there is usually no talking to allow the practitioner to focus on the passage of energy for the highest good of the client. The practitioner will then lay hands on the recipient in pre-determined positions to cover the major organs of the body.

214

The client may experience several things during the treatment: a sense of calm, heat, tingling, vibration, or nothing at all. In addition, the effects of a Reiki treatment may not be realized for several days, but will always show up when most needed. It is important to remember that Reiki treatments are not disease-specific. For instance, a goal in a Reiki treatment session isn't to cure cancer, but rather to afford the body the strength it needs to deal with its problems, the wisdom to use the energy for the best possible outcome, and to provide the courage, — emotionally, mentally, and spiritually to endure the things to come.

After the treatment, the practitioner will discuss the treatment and the experience with the recipient. In addition the practitioner may share impressions gained during the passage of hands over the body, a procedure called scanning, in which subtle energetic disturbances may be detected by the trained practitioner.

Now, I'm sure this explanation may be a bit unsatisfying for the curious, because it's hard to describe something like this without experiencing it. So, my advice to you is, if this has aroused a curiosity about Reiki, contact a Reiki practitioner and set up a treatment. I think you will find that it is an amazing complement to most any conventional therapy you may be receiving.

What are the benefits of Meditation?

We live in a stressful society. For millions of years, man has had to deal with stress. Whether we were being chased by a saber-toothed tiger, or being cut off in traffic, we have lived with stress. Our bodies have developed a finely tuned way to deal with stress. Commonly called the "fight or flight response," it has served us well for millennia. In simple terms, when we are exposed to stress, our body prepares us to either fight or flee. It does this by increasing our heart rate and blood pressure; making us breath faster to get more oxygen; dilating the pupils in our eyes so we can see better; and shifting the blood flow from our guts to our muscles to give them a strong supply of oxygen and nutrients. All of this is done to give us an advantage if we encounter the predator on our walk in the woods. For, if that were to happen, we had three choices: fight, flee, or be lunch. You see, we do not have sharp claws or teeth. We have our brain and this adaptive response.

All of that served us well in the jungle when we could expend all the adrenaline and other stress hormones fighting or fleeing. Unfortunately, we don't have those options when someone cuts us off in traffic, or when our boss yells at us, or when the bills come in and there is more month than money. In those situations, we have no constructive way to dissipate the stress, and, without a release, it accumulates, causing negative physiological effects. That is the disadvantage of this protective response in the 21st Century.

Fortunately, our Creator gave us a balancing set of responses to restore ourselves to the resting state. Called the ***relaxation response***, it reverses the effects described above: slows the heart rate, lowers blood pressure, slows down our breathing, and allows us overall to rest and recover. This response had previously been thought to be outside our conscious control. Like the stress response, it was thought to be involuntary.

Studies done by Dr. Herbert Benson, and detailed in his book **The Relaxation Response** (1975), demonstrated that through ***Transcendental Meditation***, and with practice, a person could voluntarily induce this response, and attain all the benefits. Since that time, there has been a considerable amount of research that has examined the physiologic as well as the psychological benefits of ***meditation***. Meditation

216

and its benefits fall within a category of therapies called "***Mind-Body Therapies***." These therapies acknowledge the fact that our thoughts and feelings are inseparable from our physiology. I always tell a patient that, if they don't believe it, think about what happens when they are embarrassed. They blush, a physical reaction to an emotion.

For years, this relationship has been known in many religious traditions, and the focused attention of ***prayer*** or ***meditation*** has been a part of many religious ceremonies. But meditation is not just for such purposes. As a health care provider, it is important to recognize this therapy for its value in our 21st Century stressful society.

There are two main branches of Meditation: ***concentration methods***, in which the emphasis is on focused attention directed on a specific object, like a candle, or on something rhythmic, like breathing; and ***mindfulness methods***, in which the focus is on our sensations, our surroundings, or what we are doing at the time. Although they seem dissimilar, there is some overlap. ***Mindful meditation*** presupposes an ability to concentrate on one thing at a time.

Meditation, whether concentration focused or mindful, has been shown to be beneficial in many conditions, including heart disease, hypertension, anxiety disorder, chronic pain, substance abuse, cancer, as well as a host of others. The principle behind its use is to provide a relaxation response, which, in turn, enhances healing and contributes to lower levels of stress hormones, which are destructive if left unchecked.

Meditation is not difficult to learn; actually, the principles can be taught in a matter of minutes. As would be expected, one's proficiency and benefits increase with repeated practice. I would encourage you to give it a try. There are many guided meditation CDs available that can start you off on this track. In addition, one of my favorite books on mindful meditation is, **Wherever You Go, There You Are**, by Jon Kabat-Zinn. I practice both types of meditation. Frequently I will use the concentration meditation when unwinding at the end of the day, or to begin the day in a focused way. I practice the mindful meditation when running, working in the yard, or doing household chores, like washing dishes. Great relaxation can be derived from attention to the simple details like how the water runs off the plate as you rinse it. Give it a try yourself – it might make those stressful days more bearable.

What can Yoga do for me?

Yoga is an ancient healing system that originated in India. It is founded on several core principles, including control of the body through correct posture and breathing, calming of the mind and emotions, and meditation and contemplation. The practice of yoga came to this country in the late 19th Century. After more than 100 years, American practitioners have come to realize that with consistent practice, amazing personal transformation can happen on many levels. These changes include reduced stress, enhanced feelings of well-being, improved health and energy and healing of diseases of the mind and body. While these claims may sound excessive, many students who start yoga to improve their flexibility find that over time, they find a greater understanding of their self, increased emotional growth, and spiritual enrichment.

There are many styles of yoga, and the discussion of each is beyond the scope of this publication. However, there are certain aspects that are common to each. First are the *postures*, or *asanas*. There are more than 1000 asanas in *Hatha yoga*, the type of yoga most familiar to Americans. They are designed to simultaneously bring about flexibility, strength, and balance. In addition, they promote a sense of mental and physical well-being. They also bring about the efficient functioning of the internal organs, and enhance clarity and focus of the mind, thus bringing the entire system into a state of balance.

The second aspect all forms of yoga have in common is **breathing**. **Prana** is the Sanskrit term for **life energy**. It is analogous to the term **Ki**, as defined above in the section on Reiki. In yoga, the goal is to control the breath. By controlling the ebb and flow of the breathing, one gains control over the subtle energies of the body, and in so doing gains control over the mind.

The third aspect of yoga is **meditation**. As the practitioner assumes the various positions and controls the breath, a state of heightened awareness and focused concentration occurs. As described above, the individual becomes more peaceful, stress is reduced, and the body is able to relax at a cellular level.

There are many studies that have looked at the benefits of yoga, and it is a good adjunctive therapy to be used with conventional therapies for heart disease, breathing disorders, and digestive disorders, as well as stress-related disorders. There are many teachers available, as well as training programs for people with such interests. Yoga is a fun, healthful and beneficial practice. Be forewarned, though: Yoga is physical activity, and as with any physical activity, over-enthusiasm can result in injury. However, if you work within your capabilities, and with a capable instructor, Yoga can be a wonderful addition to a health program. I recommend it wholeheartedly for people looking to add a new dimension to their health program. So, check with your physician to see if you might gain from some of the benefits of yoga.

I'd like to get off of some of my medicines. How can I do that?

This is a question I am asked all the time. Because people see me as a "Natural Physician," they presume that I use no pharmaceuticals in my practice. Nothing could be further from the truth. I believe, as I said earlier, that the best approach is the blending of Conventional and Complementary therapies. Although in most circumstances I will recommend lifestyle and non-pharmacologic remedies first, there are great benefits in the use of pharmaceuticals, especially in acute situations. In actuality, I just see myself as having more tools in my toolbox.

When someone comes to me with this question, my first response is to ask them, "Why?" Many times the answer they give is related to side effects or cost. In those situations, it is not the idea of pharmaceuticals that is the issue, and I will work with them to find an alternative pharmaceutical that is either cheaper or has fewer side effects.

When, however, the question is raised by someone who has a philosophical reason for getting off medications, the discussion is different. At that point, I mention that they were put on the medication because something in their body is out of balance. Whether that is, for example, the insulin to sugar balance in diabetics, the balance of cholesterol fractions, or the balance of their systolic and diastolic blood pressure, I call attention to the fact that that imbalance will not go away just by stopping the medications. Nor will the risk of complications from that imbalance.

Then, I ask them what they are willing to do to bring their physiology into balance. If they are not willing to make changes in their life other than stopping their medications, I caution them against doing that, but tell them I cannot elp them in this endeavor. If, however, they are willing participants, I discuss the fact that all disease is a process, not an event, and that a process has fluidity to it – that is, we can move it back and forth on a continuum.

Our goal is to move them in the direction of less disease. We may do this through lifestyle interventions such as exercise and diet, herbal remedies, mind-body therapies or a host of other interventions. I do not, however, stop their medicine until I am sure we are moving in the right direction. You see, there is a point on this continuum beyond which the process cannot be reversed by these methods alone. If, through our efforts, we find we are not able to get past that point, I remind them that all our interventions have been helpful, and may, in fact, slow down the disease and prevent further complications, but they still need the medications to control the situation.

There are those, however, that are so motivated that they are willing to do the things we decide together. For those people, this represents a chance to regain their health, as well as lower their health care costs, both now and in the future. I find this very rewarding as a physician – the opportunity to empower a patient to take charge of his/her own healthcare and future. It is one of the most gratifying things I do on a daily basis.

To understand this further, let me give you an example: A 57-year-old man comes to see me with a 15-year history of hypertension. He takes three blood pressure medications, has elevated cholesterol, borderline blood sugar, but has no known history of cardiac disease, having had a normal stress test 6 months ago. He is 40 pounds overweight for his height, has a high-stress job as an executive and does not get regular exercise. He does not smoke, but drinks three to four martinis at night to relax. He does not sleep well, and needs

221

four cups of coffee each morning to awaken. He frequently skips breakfast, eats fast food at lunch, and whatever his wife fixes for dinner. He takes no supplements, because someone once told him it was a waste of time and only caused expensive urine. He comes to me tired of the medications, which have a negative effect on his sex life and his energy level. He would like to get off the medicines, if possible.

When I meet with him, he is truly motivated, because he does not like the way he feels. We discuss the fact that he may have to give up some of the things he currently relies on to get through his day, and he agrees.

The plan we come up with together is as follows: He will slowly wean himself from his caffeine and the martinis. He will purchase a pedometer and monitor the amount of steps he puts in per day. He will begin eating breakfast and will keep a diet diary to determine the type of intake he has. He will start on a comprehensive multivitamin and mineral product, as well as some fish oil and magnesium on a daily basis. From his diet diary, we will determine what sort of nutritional counseling he may need. He is instructed in some basic meditation techniques which he will do as part of his bedtime ritual, and will monitor the quantity and quality of his sleep. We may try some melatonin to help induce sleep if necessary.

The plan is explained to him, and then he decides which parts he can implement right away, choosing the dietary and sleep issues. He elects to try the melatonin, while he learns and practices the meditation techniques, and weans the caffeine and alcohol. Two weeks later, his blood pressure is down twenty points and we drop one of his medications. He is seen every two weeks and makes great strides, growing in confidence and self-empowerment. After 6 months, he has lost 15 pounds,

222

s sleeping better, eating better, and is off two blood pressure medications. He has more energy and is enjoying life more.

While this is not an actual patient story, it is representative of what can happen when a patient who is motivated takes control and responsibility for his health. If this approach makes sense to you, discuss it with your physician, and maybe together you can accomplish great things with your health.

How do I discuss some of these things with my Doctor?

The basis of any good physician-patient relationship is strong rapport and communication. Both parties must agree that they are working toward the same goals and are partners in the therapeutic process. It is to your advantage to have a physician that you can go to for education when you have a question about your health.

Most physicians today are aware that there are different healing disciplines available to the consumer. It is mutually advantageous to you and your physician to know what your concerns are and what you, as a self-motivated consumer, would like to pursue. After all, you are partners. You must be comfortable approaching him about what you would like to investigate, why and what you hope to gain. He, in turn, must be open minded enough to hear your concerns, give you honest and objective feedback and to respect your choice. He must also be willing to educate himself about the area in which you have an interest.

This interaction should not be undersold for several reasons. First, if you feel belittled or discounted, there could be irreparable harm to your relationship. Second, if you do not tell him what you want to do, there could be potentially

223

harmful interactions between what you are doing and what he is trying to do. If he is unaware, he cannot foresee these problems. Third, there is tremendous benefit to be gained working as a team and accomplishing your goals – you are empowered, and he may gain some new information that can be useful to other patients.

Don't be afraid! It's your health we're talking about! Hopefully, through this brief overview of complementary therapies, you may discover some new ideas which might benefit you, your health or the health of someone you care about. I hope you will use these concepts in the spirit they were intended: ***Be well!***

Chapter 15

What You Need to Know About Cancer

Shobha Chitneni, MD
Sue Clarahan, RD, LD
Karen Crawford, BSN, CRNI, OCN
Faith Damewood, RN, OCN
Stefanie Dreher, RN, OCN
Pam Iverson, RN, OCN

What is Cancer?

Normally cells in our body grow and divide in an organized fashion. New cells replace old cells as the older cells die off. *Cancer* occurs when normal cells become abnormal and begin to divide and grow rapidly before older cells die. These cells can form excess tissue which may be a cancerous tumor. These cancerous tumors can occur in any tissue such as the breast, colon, or organ such as the liver, and supporting tissue in the body. Some cancers do not form tumors, as is the case with *leukemia*, which is a cancer of the blood cells.

In order to determine the type of cancer, a small amount of tissue is removed from the tumor through a needle or surgery. It is sent to a lab at which tests are performed in order to determine which cells in the body the cancer cells most closely resemble. This is how the primary cancer is identified. Cancer cells can break off and travel to other parts of the body such as the liver, bones, lung or brain. The cancer cells then begin to grow in those areas as well. When cancer spreads in this manner it is called *metastasis*. For example, if a person has breast cancer which spreads to the lung they do not have lung cancer they have *breast cancer with metastasis to the lung*. This is an important distinction to make as treatment is directed towards the primary cancer (in the organ of origin) and not to where the tumor has spread.

Seven Warning Signs of Cancer

Seven commonly recognized signs of cancer may include:
- A change in bowel or bladder habits
- A sore that does not heal
- Any unusual bleeding or discharge
- A thickening or lump in the breast or elsewhere
- Indigestion or difficulty swallowing
- Obvious change in a wart or mole
- Nagging cough or hoarseness

If you have any of these signs, it is recommended that you see your physician. There may be additional signs that do not appear on this list that require you to seek the advice of your physician.

What Are Some Ways To Prevent Cancer?

Routine Screenings and Preventative Measures
- Pap smear
- Perform monthly self breast exams
- Mammogram annually
- PSA (Prostate Specific Antigen test) annually
- Colonoscopy after age 50, then every 5-10 years
- Annual fecal occult blood test
- Have your physician inspect your skin for changes in moles, growths or sunspots
- Do not smoke or chew tobacco
- Wear sunscreen of at least SPF 20 and avoid tanning beds
- Maintain a healthy weight throughout life
- Eat a healthy diet, with an emphasis on plant foods
- Limit alcohol use to no more than 1 drink per day for women and 2 drinks per day for men
- Avoid exposure to known carcinogens such as radon, asbestos, second-hand smoke, and other workplace chemicals

- Adopt sexual practices that limit your exposure to sexually transmitted diseases, such as use of condoms, limit your sexual partners, and abstinence
- Keep appointments for annual physical and dental visits

You may have more frequent screenings based upon your family history, your lifestyle, and other pre-existing health problems.

Important Tip: You know your body better than anyone else. If something is unusual or wrong, do not delay going to the doctor to get it checked out.

What are the best meal guidelines for cancer prevention and treatment?

Many foods that help prevent cancer in the first place also seem to help us beat the disease when it has struck. According to the American Cancer Society and the American Institute for Cancer Research, try to use the following information as a template for a healthy diet:

- Eat a variety of foods, with emphasis on a plant-based diet.
- Eat plenty of fruits and vegetables. Try to eat 5 or more servings daily. Limit French fries and other fried vegetables.
- Choose whole grains and minimize refined or processed grains and sugars.
- Limit red meat to less than three ounces daily. Obtain protein from legumes, tofu, fish and poultry.
- Do not eat charred foods; meat and fish grilled over direct flames and cured and smoked meats should be consumed only occasionally.
- Use a modest amount of oil and fat. Limit saturated fats, deep-fried foods. Fat is very calorie-dense, so

227

even the healthier fats such as nuts, canola and olive oil should be used sparingly.

- Cut back on salt; limit processed foods.
- Limit alcohol to less than two drinks/day for men and one drink/day for women. A drink is equivalent to 12 oz. beer, 4 oz. wine or 1 oz. hard liquor.
- Maintain a healthy weight and exercise daily throughout life.

What Cookbooks Could You Recommend?

What Color is Your Diet? The Seven Colors of Health, by David Heber, MD., Ph.D., with Susan Bowerman, M.S., R.D., (Regan Books, 2001)

The New American Plate Cookbook, Recipes for a Healthy Weight and a Healthy Lifestyle, by the American Institute for Cancer Research, (University of California Press, 2005)

Betty Crocker's Living with Cancer Cookbook, by Betty Crocker Kitchens; Cheri Olerud editor, (Hungry Minds, 2002)

The Cancer Survival Cookbook: 200 Quick & Easy Recipes with Helpful Eating Hints, by Donna L. Weihofen, R.D., M.S., Christina Marino, M.D., MPH. (Chronimed Publishing, 1998)

The Cancer Recovery Healthy Exchanges Cookbook, by JoAnna M. Lund, (Penguin Putman Inc, 2000)

Do I Need Nutritional Supplements?

Foods, especially fruits and vegetables, contain many potentially healthy compounds, and research shows these compounds work best together, as found naturally in foods. Many people take a multivitamin and mineral supplement that provides 100% of the ***dietary reference intake (DRI)*** "for insurance." But many times people who receive a diagnosis of cancer decide to try nutritional supplements such as vitamins, minerals, herbs and herbal remedies while undergoing treatment. Research shows that these products can interfere with cancer treatment. Why is it vital that you talk to your health care team when you take any type of nutritional supplements? Nutritional supplements may cause:

- Medications not to work properly
- Medications to be processed too quickly
- Medications to be processed too slowly
- Your liver to be overwhelmed and become damaged

There is not enough research to know all of the ways that supplements might interfere with cancer medications. Some supplements can be safe and beneficial to take during treatment. Discuss these products with members of your health care team that are knowledgeable about nutritional supplements, such as a registered dietitian, registered nurse or physician. Together you and your health care team can come up with the best plan for both your medications and any nutritional supplements you'd like to take.

What Types Of Cancer Are Most Common As We Age?

According to the ***National Cancer Institute***, 60 percent of newly diagnosed cancers and 70 percent of cancer deaths occur in people over the age of 65. Several theories attribute this fact to changes that occur as we age, such as changes in our immune system, our body's ability to repair damage to our DNA, and our lifetime exposure to environmental toxins. These factors may also affect which symptoms first alert us that something is not right and also how our bodies respond to cancer treatments.

The types of cancer that are linked to aging include cancers of the breast, prostate, colon, rectum, lung, bladder, and pancreas. Early detection and early treatment are the key. It is important to have annual physical exams and screening tests and to alert your primary care physician if you develop any symptoms that concern you.

What Should I Ask The Doctor?

Good communication between you and your healthcare team is important. When a person gets a cancer diagnosis, often there is more than one doctor, i.e., surgeon, doctor administering chemotherapy or radiation therapy doctor. You can help your doctor by making a list of your questions and being honest about your lifestyle, such as smoking and/or herbal remedy use. Be as clear and as accurate as you can about reporting problems to your doctor. Make a list of questions you have and problems you experience that you wish to discuss with the doctor. For example, write down if you had nausea for three days.

Here are some questions you can ask your doctor:
- What cancer do I have?
- Has my cancer spread?
- What is the recommended treatment?
- What is the goal of treatment?
- What are my other treatment options?
- How will the treatments be given?
- How will my treatments make me feel?
- What are the side effects?
- How will the side effects be managed?
- What are the risks and benefits of my treatment?
- How will I know the treatment is working?
- How often will I have follow-up testing?
- Who should I call with questions?
- Will I see other doctors?

- Will I have restrictions in diet, work, activities, exercise or sexual relations?
- If my treatment doesn't work, what are my other options?
- How do I get a second opinion?

Important Tip: Don't be afraid to ask the doctor to explain something again to you. You may be overwhelmed by what the doctor is saying due to anxiety and fear of a new cancer diagnosis. It may be helpful to bring a family member or friend to help you remember what the doctor is saying.

What Tests Will Be Necessary?

There are many different tests or a combination of tests that may be used to determine what is wrong with you. Here is a list of the most common diagnostic tests in alphabetical order:

- Biopsy
  A *biopsy* is removing a piece of the suspected tissue and sending it to be looked at under a microscope. This is one way cancer is diagnosed. There are different types of biopsies that your doctor will explain to you.

- Blood Tests
  In some cases when certain types of cancer are suspected, there are specific *blood tests* that can be done to help determine the probable origin of the cancer. These tests are called *tumor markers*. They can show an increase with the presence of cancer. They can also help in monitoring treatment by showing an increase or decrease in the levels. Some examples of tumor markers are CA19-9 and CEA, which can be tumor markers for colorectal cancer.

- Bone Scan
  A ***bone scan*** takes images of the skeletal system. It is much more sensitive than a plain X-ray. The main reason a bone scan is done is to detect the spread of cancer to the bones.

- Bronchoscopy
  In a ***bronchoscopy***, a thin flexible lighted tube is inserted into the nose or mouth to view the ***voice box (larynx)***, the ***throat (trachea)***, and ***lungs***. Tissue can be obtained during this test to help diagnose abnormalities.

- CAT Scan (Computed Axial Tomography); CT Scan (Computed Tomography)
  A ***CT scan*** produces three-dimensional pictures of your body so doctors get a clear view of changes. It can be ordered with or without contrast. Contrast is a material that can be given orally, IV (intravenous) or rectally. Contrast helps highlight certain tissue for better images.

- Colonoscopy
  In a ***colonoscopy***, a flexible, lighted scope is inserted into the rectum and passed through the entire ***colon*** to the ***cecum***. The doctor will be able to see and take pictures of any abnormalities. The doctor can also take samples of tissue during this test.

- MRI (Magnetic Resonance Imaging)
  Magnetic Resonance Imaging, or ***MRI***, is a diagnostic technique that uses a magnetic field to produce pictures of structures inside the body.

- MUGA (Multiple Gated Acquisition)
  MUGA is a painless heart scan to evaluate the

condition of the heart. It is not done to diagnose but to be sure the heart is strong enough to withstand chemotherapy drugs that may damage the heart.

- PET Scan (Positive Emission Tomography)
  A *PET scan* is an imaging technique that uses positively charged particles (radioactive positrons) to detect subtle changes in the body's metabolism and chemical activities. A PET scan provides a color-coded image of the body's function, rather than its structure.

- Spinal Tap (Lumbar Puncture)
  In a *spinal tap*, a needle is placed into the low-back area into the spinal column to obtain fluid for testing. It can determine if cancer is in the central nervous system. It can also be done to inject therapeutic medication.

- Ultrasound
  In an *ultrasound* exam, a wand or probe is rubbed over an area with a lubricating gel that produces high frequency sound waves, which form an image. It can detect abnormalities.

- Urine Tests
  There are different tests that can be done with *urine*. Since urine is a waste product, an increase or decrease in certain values in urine can indicate kidney, bladder, or other organ disease.

- X-ray
  In an *X-ray*, a high-energy electromagnetic wave is used to take pictures of your body to view soft tissue and bone structure. It can detect larger tumors and abnormalities.

What Are My Treatment Options?

There are several methods for treating cancer. Some of the treatment options are ***surgery***, ***chemotherapy***, ***radiation therapy***, ***hormone therapy***, ***biologic therapy***, ***clinical trials*** and ***observation***. Your doctor will discuss which treatment option is best for you based upon the type and location of the cancer, the stage of the disease, your age and your general health. You may receive one method of treatment or a combination of several methods to treat your cancer.

- Surgery

  Surgery is used to remove the tumor. Tissue around the tumor and nearby lymph nodes may also be removed during the operation.

- Chemotherapy

  Chemotherapy medicines are drugs used to kill cancer cells and to prevent cancer from spreading. Chemotherapy changes the ability of cancer cells to divide and grow. You may receive one drug or a combination of several different drugs to treat your cancer. Chemotherapy is given either into a vein (***intravenous*** or ***IV***), taken in pill form, or given in an injection. Chemotherapy may be given in your doctor's office, hospital, clinic or even at home.

- Radiation Therapy

  Radiation uses a concentrated form of energy to destroy or damage cancer cells. It can be given externally in the form of X-ray beams, or radioactive substances may be placed inside the body or directly into the tumor itself.

- Hormone Therapy

  Hormone therapy is used against certain cancers that depend on hormones for their growth. Hormone therapy keeps cancer cells from getting or using the hormones they need. This treatment may include the use of drugs that stop the production of certain hormones or that change the way they work.

- Biologic Therapy or Immunotherapy
  Our immune system normally recognizes and fights off foreign substances in our bodies. ***Biologic agents*** are used to help boost the immune response to fight and destroy cancer cells.

- Clinical Trials
  In certain cases, you may be asked to participate in a clinical trial. ***Clinical trials*** (research studies) offer important treatment options for many people with cancer. Research studies evaluate promising new therapies and answer scientific questions. The goal of such trials is to find treatments that are more effective in controlling cancer with fewer side effects.

- Observation
  Occasionally, if you have a small, slow-growing type of cancer, you and your physician may decide that ***observation*** is the right action for you. Your healthcare team would monitor your disease regularly. You would have the option of treatment if the cancer would grow or spread.

What Life Style Changes Will Occur?

After the diagnosis of cancer, you may experience some ***lifestyle changes***. These changes can affect your quality of life and include physical, emotional and social changes.

Physical changes may include:
- Temporary hair loss
- Temporary side effects of chemotherapy including nausea, heartburn, mouth sores, decreased appetite, constipation and diarrhea
- Pain and fatigue
- Changes in your body from surgery or radiation

Social changes may include:
- Changes in your work schedule or job due to treatment or doctor appointments
- Not going out to eat or socialize as often due to fatigue or low blood counts
- Depending on friends and family to run errands, help you at home and prepare your meals
- Changes in your relationship with family, friends and co-workers

Emotional changes may include:
- Feelings of anger and fear
- Feelings of sadness or depression
- Feelings of uncertainty or anxiety
- Feeling like you have lost control

Important Tip: It is important to know your health care team is available to help you understand these changes and provide resources for you and your family to use during this time.

If Cancer Comes Back

Many people believe that if they survive 5 years without a recurrence of cancer, they are cancer-free, but the fact remains that cancer can recur at any time. If your cancer recurs:
- You may experience feelings of fear and/or anger

- You may go through many of the same tests you did when you were first diagnosed
- You may have surgery, chemotherapy, and/or radiation therapy again

Important tip: Your support networks are very important in coping with the recurrence of cancer. Your health care team will help you in getting the support you need.

What Support Options are Available?

One of the most important things that you can do if you are diagnosed with cancer is build your *support network*. Your support network may include family members, friends, persons from your religious/spiritual institution as well as those you met from support groups.

Some of the ways your support network can help you include:

- Coming with you to appointments
- Taking notes when you talk to the doctor and/or nurses
- Listening to your concerns
- Assisting with housework and cooking duties
- Running errands

Your treatment center may have a *social worker* on staff or can get you in touch with a social worker who can help you obtain some of the following services:

- Cancer information
- Counseling
- Medical treatment decisions
- Prevention and early detection
- Home health care
- Hospice care
- Rehabilitation

- Advocacy
- Financial assistance
- Transportation
- Housing/lodging assistance
- Insurance information

There are many national organizations that are dedicated to providing support for cancer patients and their families. Call the *American Cancer Society* in your area for a complete list. Information on local support resources may be obtained through a variety of sources:

- Physician's office, treatment center or hospital
- Public library
- Religious institutions
- Local or county government agencies, such as the Area Agency on Aging

Important tip: Ask for help if you need it. Don't be afraid or ashamed to ask for assistance. Having a cancer diagnosis can be very difficult, which is why it is so important to use your support network to help ease some of your burdens and allow you to focus on your treatment and recovery.

What Websites Could You Recommend?

There are many resources and organizations that offer information and support at no charge for patients, their families and health care professionals. The following is a list of websites that contain general information regarding cancer and its treatment.

American Cancer Society
www.cancer.org
Source of news, information, and support

American Dietetic Association
www.eatright.org
Source of nutrition news and information

American Society of Clinical Oncology
www.asco.org
Information for patients, doctors and scientists

Cancer Guide
www.cancerguide.org
Helps with finding answers to your questions about cancer, and guidance with questions that you need to ask

CancerCare
www.cancercare.org
Information for patients and on-line support groups

CancerConsultants
www.cancerconsultants.com
Provides up-to-date information on the treatment and prevention of cancer, patients and professionals

CancerLinks
www.cancerlinks.org
Provides a comprehensive list of links for different kinds of cancers

Cancer Nutrition Information
www.cancernutritioninfo.com Helps people understand the link between nutrition and cancer

Cancer Research and Prevention Foundation
www.preventcancer.org
Group dedicated to cancer prevention through research and education

Consumer Labs
www.consumerlabs.com
Mission: To identify the best quality health and nutrition products through independent testing

International Cancer Alliance for Research and Education
www.icare.org
Provides focused, user-friendly cancer information

Leukemia Lymphoma Society
www. leukemia&lymphomasociety.org
Provides information on blood-related cancers, education, patient services and support services

National Cancer Institute Cancer Information
www.cancer.gov
Service: Free resources and educational materials on all cancer types

National Comprehensive Cancer Network
www.nccn.com
Provides state-of-the-art care to patients, advances research on prevention, and enhances the effectiveness of cancer care delivery

Oncology Nursing Society
www.ONS.org
Information on cancer prevention

Chapter 16

An Overview of Rheumatic Illnesses
David B. Staub, MD

What is the immune system and how is it related to arthritis?

The *immune system* is made of white cells and molecules such as *antibodies* and *cytokines* which help the *white cells* communicate with one another. The elements of the immune system are responsible for inflammation. The classical features of inflammation in tissues are redness, warmth, and swelling.

The immune system has three primary responsibilities. One is to recognize infectious microbes and kill them. Another is to recognize cancer when it develops and kill it. A third responsibility is to recognize the individual's "self" tissues and not disturb or attack these tissues. If the immune system fails in any one of these regards, the individual develops health problems.

In the first instance are problems with infection such as pneumonia. In the second instance cancer can develop. And in the third instance autoimmune disease can develop. *Autoimmune diseases* are *inflammatory rheumatic diseases*. Examples include *rheumatoid arthritis*, *lupus*, and *vasculitis*. Inflammatory rheumatic diseases can include inflammation in many different parts of the body. Organ systems as varied as the heart, gastrointestinal tract, lung, skin, eye, joints, or muscles can become inflamed. When the joints are inflamed, we call this *arthritis*.

How does osteoarthritis differ from rheumatoid arthritis?

Rheumatoid arthritis is caused by the immune system

gone awry, attacking the individual's joints. This can give rise to the classical features of inflammation which are redness, warmth, pain, and swelling at given joints. ***Osteoarthritis*** is more a mechanical problem and is due to cartilage abnormalities or how the joint mechanically functions; most of the features of inflammation (redness, swelling, and warmth) are not present. Many of the new treatments becoming available are designed to quiet down the inflammation of rheumatoid arthritis. These treatments, however, do not work in ***osteoarthritis***.

What are NSAIDs (nonsteroidal antiinflammatory drugs)?

The original ***NSAID (nonsteroidal antiinflammatory drug)*** is ***aspirin,*** which was isolated in 1897. A derivative was later developed called ***indomethacin (Indocin),*** and since then many other derivatives have been developed and marketed. These drugs also include ***sulindac (Clinoril), nabumetone (Relafen), salsalate (Disalcid), ibuprofen (Motrin, Advil), and naproxen (Naprosyn, Aleve),*** among many others. The main side effects of the NSAID's are that they cause peptic ulcer disease and sometimes kidney problems. The most recently developed sub-family of NSAID's is the ***COX-2 selective agents***. These drugs were introduced because they were considered to have a lower risk of peptic ulcer disease than traditional nonsteroidal antiinflammatory drugs. The first of these drugs was ***celecoxib (Celebrex)***. ***Rofecoxib (Vioxx)*** and ***valdecoxib (Bextra)*** were later introduced; however, they are no longer on the market due to concern about cardiovascular risks. Celecoxib remains on the market. None of the traditional NSAID's or newer COX-2 drugs has ever been demonstrated to halt joint damage over time. The sole reason to use these drugs is for pain reduction.

What is cortisone?

Cortisone was first given to a human being in 1948 and is similar to the body's *cortisol,* which is made by the *adrenal gland*. These compounds are called *adrenocorticosteroids* and include synthetic *prednisone*, *prednisolone*, and *dexamethasone*, among others. These drugs are potent antiinflammatory drugs that have profound effects on inflammation caused by the immune system. The drugs have use in many forms of inflammatory arthritis as well as many other inflammatory conditions – for example, *sarcoidosis* and *asthma*.

What are the Disease Modifying Drugs (DMARD's)?

Certain *disease-modifying drugs (DMARD's)* have been available for over 50 years. These are drugs which have been found to have an effect on the immune system. Currently the most widely used of these drugs is *methotrexate (Rheumatrex)*. Other examples are *azathioprine (Imuran), cyclophosphamide (Cytoxan), mycophenolate (CellCept), sulfasalazine (Azulfidine)*, and *hydroxychloroquine (Plaquenil)*. These drugs have a strong effect on the immune system but are slow-acting drugs. Thus, three to six months of continuous use must pass before the individual begins to feel a favorable effect from these agents. Likewise, when the drug is stopped, often three to six more months must pass before a flare-up recurs. These drugs have been tested in rheumatoid arthritis and many of these agents have been shown to slow down joint damage over time. Some of these drugs are also used in other inflammatory rheumatic diseases such as *lupus* and *vasculitis*.

What are the Biologic Response Modifiers (BRM's)?

The *biologic response modifiers* are agents that have an effect on the immune system and its activity. The first group of BRM's used in treating patients with rheumatic disease includes the *TNF blockers*. These include *infliximab (Remicade), etanercept (Enbrel)*, and *adalimumab (Humira)*. *TNF (tumor necrosis factor)* is a substance called a *cytokine* which is produced by the white blood cells to communicate with one another. TNF levels are much higher than normal in people with rheumatoid arthritis, and the TNF blockers are designed to block the effects of the excess TNF. In so doing, the arthritis becomes less active and less prone to causing damage to joints over time.

Another BRM is *anakinra (Kineret)*; this agent blocks the effects of a cytokine called *interleukin 1*. Two recently introduced BRM's are *abatacept (Orencia)* and *rituximab (Rituxan)*. The first of these blocks the direct communication between certain white blood cells. The second of these depletes the body of a certain group of white cells called *B-lymphocytes*. The result of using each of these various agents is to lessen the inflammation in joints.

What can be done to slow down or halt the worsening of osteoarthritis?

No pharmaceutical or other measures have been shown to prevent worsening of *osteoarthritis* over a time. Although *glucosamine* and/or *chondroitin* have been touted for this, the science supporting these agents is lacking. Studies have shown, however, that weight loss will definitely slow down the worsening of osteoarthritis of the knee. Thus, if a person is overweight and has arthritis of weight-bearing joints, this individual should make every effort to get down to his or her ideal body weight.

What over-the-counter supplements are used for rheumatoid arthritis?

Omega-3 fatty acids found in fish oils have been shown to be of benefit when used in large doses in rheumatoid arthritis. Studies have demonstrated that in established rheumatoid arthritis, high doses do improve the symptoms of rheumatoid arthritis to a mild degree.

What over-the-counter supplements are used for osteoarthritis?

Glucosamine and *chondroitin* have been promoted for use in osteoarthritis. This is based on many largely European-controlled studies which have been done over the past 25 years. The largest, best-designed study, however, was recently published in America, sponsored by the *National Institute of Health,* and this showed no significant benefit by using glucosamine alone. Of the various groups studied, the only group shown to have any benefit was the glucosamine plus chondroitin combination group when used in patients with severe osteoarthritis. The milder osteoarthritic groups did not have benefit with this combination or the glucosamine or chondroitin used alone. One must remember that this American study and the earlier European studies looked at pain reduction. Joint space cartilage loss over time has seldom been tested in the studies done and thus the claim that glucosamine and/or chondroitin can "repair" cartilage is unfounded. These supplements tend to be expensive and the most recent, best-done study indicates no convincing benefit.

On what grounds is a given treatment recommended?

When treating arthritis patients, we like to choose our treatments based on the results of scientific studies. The standard controlled study starts with a group of patients with a particular illness – for example, rheumatoid arthritis. The

245

patients are then randomly assigned into either a ***treatment group*** (the group to receive the experimental drug) or a ***control group*** (the group to receive a ***placebo*** treatment). Neither the patients nor the physicians involved know who is in which group (this is referred to as a double-blinded experiment) and only the pharmacist has a record of which patient is in which group. Baseline studies are obtained such as laboratory tests, X-rays, or MRI scans on the individual patients. The patients then begin taking either the experimental drug or the placebo (whichever a given patient has been randomized to receive) for a predetermined period of time – for example, 6 or 12 months. Throughout the period and after that time frame, various measurements are taken to quantify the degree of pain and finally X-rays and other studies are often taken at the end. An individual subject is then assessed as to whether this person gets better, gets worse or stays the same. Then the pharmacist cracks the code and the patients are identified as to whether they had received the placebo or the experimental medication. The patients who received the experimental drug are then pooled together and compared to the patients who received the placebo. If the experimental drug group in general has done better statistically than the control group, and if these results were unlikely to have occurred by chance alone, then the treatment is considered to have merit.

If a number of such double-blind, randomized, placebo-controlled studies are done and show the same results, ultimately the drug is accepted to have scientifically-proven merit. Unfortunately, this process is very time-consuming and expensive and is done reliably only for what are categorized as "drugs" by the FDA. No requirements for such testing exist with "supplements." Thus with a given supplement one generally cannot make convincing claims about its effectiveness (or safety). Often supplements are used based on folklore and intuition but not science.

What other supplements have been promoted for arthritis treatment?

Dimethyl sulfoxide (DMSO) is a derivative from wood pulp which has been promoted to improve osteoarthritis pain when applied locally to the skin over joints. *S-adenosylmethionine (SAMe)* is a compound which occurs in all living cells and has been again commercially available by prescription in Europe since 1975. *Cetyl myristoleate* is a new agent which has also been promoted for osteoarthritis. Scientific studies designed to test the usefulness and safety of these supplements are sparse and some are flawed statistically, and thus these agents cannot be recommended for arthritis.

Does smoking have an effect on rheumatoid arthritis?

Yes. Twin studies from United Kingdom demonstrated that in monozygotic (identical) twins, the twin who smoked had a higher chance of developing rheumatoid arthritis than did the non-smoking twin. More recently, studies have shown that a newly recognized antibody called *anti-cyclic citrullinated peptide antibody* is associated with more serious arthritis and is more likely to occur in smoking individuals than non-smoking individuals.

What is an antinuclear antibody?

All human beings have antibodies; without antibodies we could not fight microbes and remain healthy. In the laboratory, when one of the antibodies reacts against the nucleus of a cell, it is called an *antinuclear antibody (ANA)*. Many individuals who have completely good health will have an ANA; thus, this does not always signify a health problem. Many years ago the ANA was first discovered, and initially researchers could get a clue about whether an ANA was significant by how the ANA looked under the microscope. To test this, first cells are placed on a slide, and then the patient's

247

blood is exposed to these cells. After additional measures are taken, one can directly observe, with a microscope, a pattern produced by the antibody attaching itself to the nucleus of a cell. Certain patterns suggest certain illnesses. For example, a speckled pattern suggests *scleroderma* and a pattern around the rim of the nucleus suggests *lupus*.

As the technology improved, researchers began to identify the particular constituent of the nucleus against which the antibody was directed. These specific antibodies help tremendously in identifying patients whose ANA's may be important. For example, a certain antibody (against DNA) within the nucleus correlates strongly with lupus. Another antibody (called *anti-centromere antibody*) correlates strongly with a certain type of scleroderma. These antibody tests can be quite useful in helping to sort out which type of rheumatic illness a given patient has.

What is scleroderma?

Scleroderma (also known as systemic sclerosis) is a condition in which too much fibrous tissue accumulates in the body. One of the results of this is thickened, "hide-bound" skin. Almost all individuals with scleroderma experience *Raynaud's phenomenon.* An episode of Raynaud's will typically occur in the hands or feet when exposed to cold temperatures; first these sites will become white and painful, then red and/or blue upon re-warming. In some cases of scleroderma, internal organs such as the lung, heart, kidney and the gastrointestinal tract can also be impaired by too much fibrous tissue deposition.

What is the test for lupus?

The test for *lupus* is a thorough evaluation by a *rheumatologist*. Many patients are referred to a rheumatologist due to a positive ANA; however, a majority f these patients, in fact, do not have lupus. The antinuclear ntibody (ANA) indeed is present in 98% of patients who ltimately are shown to have lupus. At least several other eatures must be present to confidently assign the diagnosis f lupus. These features include the presence of *mouth ores, arthritis, pleurisy, certain types of skin rashes* (often /orse in the sun), *low blood counts, protein in the urine* and ertain *neurological problems*. If a given patient has only a ositive ANA but none of these other features, this individual /ill not be given the diagnosis of lupus.

Vhat causes gout?

out is caused by uric acid. This molecule is a normal reakdown product in the life cycle of human cells. In some atients this will accumulate to high levels which tend to leposit out in joints and other soft tissues. The deposits tend o occur in cooler parts of the body such as the feet or hands. ertain risk factors make an individual more likely to have gout. These include the use of diuretics (water pills) and xcess use of alcohol. Gout often strikes men generally at or)eyond the middle ages of life and postmenopausal women. 'remenopausal women virtually never get gout. The long-erm management of gout centers on the reduction of the)lood uric acid level to make sure this level is consistently)elow 6.2 mg/dL, generally between 5.0 and 6.0 mg/dL. A number of traditional medications have been available for many years to do this (*probenecid* and *allopurinol*), and a new drug will soon be released by the FDA for this purpose *febuxostat*). When managing a sudden attack of gout, a number of other medications are used.

What is fibromyalgia?

Fibromyalgia is categorized as a rheumatic illness and consists of pain perceived in the muscles, generally in the /icinity of the shoulders, elbows, neck, back, hips, and knees.

249

This illness occurs more often in women than men and the onset is generally between 30 and 45 years of age. Many theories about the origin of this illness exist. Past research on the muscles and nerves has proven to be fruitless and most of the current research focuses on the central nervous system (brain). Childhood emotional trauma in some cases has played a role in later development of fibromyalgia; in other patients no such history exists. The treatments which have proven to be most successful have been physical therapy, stretching and aerobic exercises, and medications to deepen the sleep.

What is myofascial pain and how is it related to bursitis and tendonitis?

Myofascial tissue is made up of the fibrous planes which separate one muscle component from the next and the myofascial planes of tissue coalesce to form tendons *(See Figure 1)*. The muscle/tendon unit is responsible for moving the joint. Myofascial pain occurs within broad areas of muscle (such as the upper back on toward the shoulder).

Myofascial pain, *bursitis* and *tendonitis* are similar to one another. *Soft tissue pain* is the common feature in each case (in contrast to pain from the bone or joint). Bursitis is pain resulting from the *bursa*. The body has over 150 of these fluid-filled sacs in various places, generally near joints. These fluid-filled bursae exist to allow moving parts near joints to move more efficiently. *Tendonitis* is pain resulting from a tendon. The treatment for these three conditions (bursitis, tendonitis, and myofascial pain) is similar and involves physical therapy, pain relievers, and anti-inflammatories, as well as modifications of any aggravating factors.

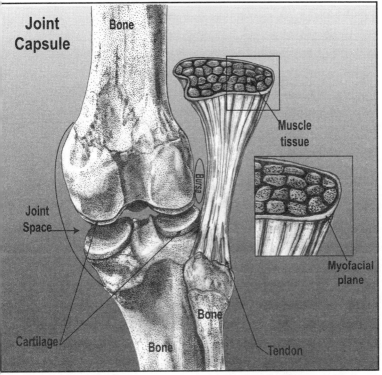

Figure 1. Joint Capsule with tendon and muscle components

Readers experiencing difficulties from any of the symptoms listed in this chapter are encouraged to consult their primary care physician or a rheumatologist.

Chapter 17

Erectile Dysfunction and the Golden Age
Ghassoub Harb, MD, FACS

Population statisticians project that the percentage of men in the United States who are over age 65 and over age 85 is expected to continue to increase over the next 50 years. This is clearly related to tremendous advances in cardiovascular care, which place a lot of challenge for the other specialties to catch up in caring for aging patients. One of the most significant challenges faced by men over the age of 65 is *erectile dysfunction*, or *impotence*.

What is Erectile Dysfunction (ED)?

ED is simply described as the inability to achieve or maintain an erection suitable for sexual intercourse. Impotence affects 30 million American men or about 10% of the entire male population and 35% of the men over the age of 40. However, **impotence is a treatable problem, one which is NOT the inevitable consequence of aging.**

In a national survey conducted for *AARP* (*American Association of Retired Persons*) of 639 men age 45 years and older, only 10% of the respondents reported seeking or receiving treatment to improve sexual function. Only half of the men (5%) who had sought treatment had tried or were using Viagra.

How does an erection occur?

An *erection* is created when the male is sexually aroused. The *penis* fills with blood, much like a tire fills with air. The blood is pumped into the penis and not allowed out, and the more blood that is pumped in, the firmer the erection.

The reasons for lack of erections are either the lack of appropriate filling or emptying of the penis. Because the nervous system controls the arteries and veins, psychological problems can cause emptying of the penis at unwanted times. At one time it was felt that psychological causes were the most important, but we have come to realize that they are actually in a significant minority. The major causes of impotence today are diabetes, atherosclerosis or hardening of the arteries and impotence following radical pelvic surgery. Other causes include spinal cord injuries, hormonal problems, and multiple sclerosis. The abuse of drugs, alcoholism and smoking can interfere with normal erections, and well over 200 different prescription medications can cause impotence as a side effect.

How common is ED in elderly patients?

Older people may have a misconception that ED symptoms are a natural part of aging. Others may believe their symptoms are not severe enough to discuss with their healthcare provider or may be embarrassed to bring up the subject. Additionally, individuals may not be aware that treatment is available. The percentage of those patients complaining of "complete" ED remained fairly stable over the various age groups. A simple way to calculate the prevalence of complete ED above the age of 40 is by subtracting 35% from the age. For example, if you are 75 years old, the chance of complete ED is 75 years minus 35% = 40 % chance of having complete ED at the age of 75.

How do we make the diagnosis?

The diagnosis of impotence can be made by any physician. Despite the fact that more than 80% of patients expect their doctors to "ask the question" about impotence, unfortunately only 23% of doctors do! A complete history and physical along with some psychological screening and occasionally an evaluation of the hormone levels are important. Other tests may include blood tests to check the kidney function, PSA to check for prostate cancer, and fasting blood sugar to check for diabetes. Other studies include evaluation of nerve function and blood flow measurements to the penis using Doppler ultrasound. Some additional tests are invasive and expensive. While the results are often enlightening, they rarely change the options for treatment. A simple, self-administered sexual activity questionnaire (SHIM) is available at your physician's office. I encourage you to ask for one.

Does smoking increase the risk for developing ED?

A study by McVary and colleagues found that there is an association between smoking and ED. According to the analysis, the risk of moderate or complete ED was increased two-fold by cigarette smoking.

What are other risk factors for developing ED?

Other risk factors for developing erectile dysfunction include:
- Severe depression   90%
- CVD   70 %
- Multiple sclerosis   71%
- Diabetes   30-60%
- Hepatic failure   25-70%
- Chronic renal failure   40%
- Radical prostatectomy (RRP)   57 %
- Radiation therapy   40%
- RRP, with bilateral nerve sparing   20%
- Medications side effect   15-20 %

Major Risk Factors for ED: Chronic Diseases

Chronic Disease	Fold Increase ED risk
Diabetes	× 4.1 Fold Increase ED risk
Prostate disease	× 2.9 Fold Increase ED risk
Peripheral vascular disease	× 2.6 Fold Increase ED risk
Cardiac problems	× 1.8 Fold Increase ED risk
Hyperlipidemia	× 1.7 Fold Increase ED risk
Hypertension	× 1.6 Fold Increase ED risk

The flu before the fever! Could ED be an early sign of cardiovascular disease?

The small diameter of the penile vasculature suggests that the progression of *atherosclerosis* (blockage in the vessels) may lead to symptoms, including ED, earlier in this area than in the major vessels involved in coronary artery disease, stroke, and peripheral vascular disease.

Food for thought: The facts below indicate the significance of ED as a possible indicator of other health challenges and reinforce the need to share ED concerns with your doctor:

- 40% of men who sought ED treatment had significant coronary occlusions (blockages).
- 57% of men who had coronary bypass surgery reported ED before the surgery.
- 60% of men with ED and no coronary artery disease (CAD) had abnormal cholesterol levels; most had penile artery disease.

- 60% of men who were hospitalized for a myocardial infarction (MI) experienced ED before being hospitalized for the MI.

What are some shared risk factors for Erectile Dysfunction and Cardiovascular Disease?

- Hypertension
- Diabetes
- Dyslipidemia
- Sedentary life style
- Age
- Gender (Male)
- Obesity
- Smoking
- Depression

What types of medical treatment for ED are available?

A wide range of medical treatments for ED exists, including:

- Erectile dysfunction medications (such as Viagra, Levitra and Cialis)
- The homeopathic medication Yohimbe
- Hormone replacement therapy (HRT)
- Self-injection therapy
- Vacuum erection device
- Penile prostheses
- Vascular reconstructive surgery

Viagra, Levitra and Cialis

Because sexual activity can be demanding on the heart, you may want to talk to your doctor about your cardiovascular health before using these pills; they are neither hormones nor an aphrodisiac. All three of the approved *erectile dysfunction drugs* (*Viagra, Levitra* and *Cialis*) are similar in action. They are members of a family of drugs called ***PDE5 Inhibitors***. They block an enzyme that causes an erection to go flaccid (phosphodiesterase-5), keeping the blood supply to the penis stronger. Although these drugs are similar in action, their dose, onset of action time and duration of action differ. Viagra was the first PDE5 inhibitor on the market, followed by Cialis and Levitra.

What is the most effective way to take these pills?

- Take Viagra or Levitra one hour prior to engaging in sexual activity; these pills usually are effective for four hours.
- Better to take Viagra or Levitra on an empty stomach (three hours without food), because high-fat meals may take the pill longer to produce the desired effect.
- Take Cialis two hours prior to engaging in sexual activity; Cialis usually is effective for 36 hours. Cialis is usually not affected by high-fat meals; therefore, you can take it any time.
- Learn to relax; stress and anxiety can kill arousal.
- Moderate your alcohol consumption.
- If you experience any side effects, discuss it with your doctor.
- Foreplay and proper stimulation are a must! If you take any pills without receiving any sexual stimulation, it would be unlikely that an erection would occur.
- Patience and patience! If no prohibiting side effects, try it again (however, not within 24 hours). There needs to be at least six to eight attempts to call it a "failure."
- If you fail at least six attempts, or have side effects, you can ask your doctor to try the next drug in line (you might respond to a different one).

- If you have an erection that lasts more than three to four hours, inform your doctor.
- Do not combine different pills at the same time or use in combination with penile injection.
- Ask your doctor if you have any questions or concerns.
- Ask your doctor if the drug will interact with any of your medications.
- If you develop chest pain, **ALERT** your health care provider (EMS, Emergency Room, etc.) that you are taking Viagra, Levitra or Cialis, and when you last took it.
- **CAUTION: Do NOT take these pills without consulting with your doctor.**

Viagra, Levitra and Cialis Side Effects Reported by ≥ 2% of Patients.

Side Effects	Sildenafil Viagra	Vardenafil Levitra	Tadalafil Cialis
Headache	16 %	15 %	15 %
Flushing	10 %	11 %	3 %
Runny Nose		9 %	
Nasal congestion	4 %		3 %
Upset stomach	7 %	4 %	10 %
Abnormal vision	3 %		
Sinusitis		3 %	
Flu syndrome		3 %	
Diarrhea	3 %		
Back pain			6 %
Muscle pain			3 %

When is it important NOT to take Viagra, Levitra or Cialis?

Although these medications can be effective when taken as described above, there are times when they are contraindicated. Do NOT take these medications if you:

- Are taking any form of nitrates, either regularly or intermittently. When nitrate administration is deemed medically necessary in a life-threatening situation, at least 24 hours should elapse after the last dose of Viagra and Levitra and 48 hours for Cialis before nitrate use is considered.
- Use recreational drugs called "***Poppers***," like ***amyl nitrate*** and ***butyl nitrate***.

What is Yohimbe and how does it work?

Yohimbe, a medication made from the bark of a tree that grows in India and Africa, acts on the nervous system and may also have some effect on increasing the male libido. It is considered ***homeopathic*** by medical doctors — that is, no definite uses are proven — and it is reasonably safe with uncommon side effects such as mild dizziness, nervousness, headaches and nausea. Some studies have suggested that 10% to 20% of men will respond to the treatment with Yohimbe. It is necessary to take the medicine for a full two months before knowing whether it is going to work.

What is Hormone Replacement Therapy (HRT) and how does it work?

Testosterone levels can be measured by the physician at the initial evaluation. Use of the hormone ***testosterone*** can be effective in men whose production of male hormones is low. However, testosterone injections, patches or gels do not really help men who do not have low levels. Testosterone replacement can stimulate the growth of prostate tissue, which can lead to difficulty emptying the

260

bladder. Testosterone cannot be used in patients with known or suspected prostate cancer, as the cancer could grow more rapidly. Other less-common side effects of testosterone use include liver injury and increased blood pressure. Men who take testosterone regularly can become infertile.

What is self-injection therapy?

Self-injection therapy, which has been used since the early 1980s, involves the patient or his partner giving an injection of medication directly into the side of the penis to create an erection. The erection created is a natural one and usually begins 5 to 15 minutes after the injection. Not all patients respond to this type of treatment, but those that do should develop an erection that lasts anywhere from 30 to 90 minutes. The injections are given with a tiny needle and use very small amounts of medicine. The injections are relatively painless and are easily taught to the patients in one or two visits with the doctor.

Several medications are available for self-injection, including *prostaglandin E1*, such as *Caverjet®*, as a single agent, or in combination with *papaverine hydrochloride*, or *phentolamine*. Each of these medicines achieves erections by causing increased blood flow into the penis through the tiny arteries, and also by decreasing the outflow of blood from the penile veins. Considerable experience has been obtained by urologists over the past decade, and these drugs are considered safe for self-injection therapy.

What are the risks of self-injection therapy?

All medications have some potential risks and side effects, and risks do exist with all of these drugs and the injections. These may include the possibility of bleeding or bruising from the injection, as well as the small chance of infection. One of the more common risks includes the development of a *prolonged erection* or *priapism* (more than four hours), which might require a trip back to the physician or to the emergency room. Not all patients are candidates for self-injection therapy.

What are vacuum devices and how do they work?

The *vacuum erection device* is a simple mechanical tool which allows a man, without the use of medications, to develop an erection which is suitable for sexual intercourse. Erections are created when blood is trapped in the penis much like air is trapped in an inflated tire. The more air that is placed into the tire, the firmer the tire becomes. Likewise, the more blood trapped temporarily in the penis, the firmer the erection. The vacuum erection device works by bringing more blood into the penis and then trapping it. The erection can be used for up to 25 to 30 minutes. While serious injuries are rare, bruising is not uncommon and ejaculation can be painful if the tension ring placed around the base of the penis is too tight. The device can usually be tried in the office at no charge. Occasionally this method has been used for *penile rehabilitation* following prostate surgery.

What are penile prostheses and how do they work?

One of the treatment options for erectile dysfunction is the placement of a *penile prosthesis*, prosthetic inner tubes within the penis which mimics the inflation process and creates an erection. Penile implants were first used in the 1970s, and as time went on, further advances occurred.

Hundreds of thousands of men throughout the world have been successfully treated with penile implants. There is a 90%+ success rate when both partners are informed of the nature and limitations of the prosthesis. However, despite the very high rate of satisfaction, less than 4% of patients gree to have a penile implant. Today there are three types of penile prostheses: the semi-rigid implant, the inflatable implant and a self-contained inflatable implant. The newer prostheses are very reliable, and the chance of mechanical failure is very low.

What is Vascular Reconstructive Surgery?

Vascular reconstructive surgery is technically difficult, relatively expensive, and includes complications of nerve damage and scar tissue formation. Given the relatively low success rate, along with the technical difficulty and expense of this type of procedure, vascular reconstructive surgery has not been accepted widely.

What does NOT work as a treatment for ED?

At this point, there is no evidence that nutritional supplements or vitamins have any significant bearing on sexual performance. The Food and Drug Administration has currently banned the sale or advertising of all nonprescription products for the treatment of male impotence because none had been scientifically shown to be effective.

What can I do to help my sex life be more fulfilling?

- Stop smoking
- Limit or avoid alcohol
- Follow a healthy diet
- Exercise regularly
- Get adequate sleep
- Improve communications with your partner
- Talk to your doctor about checking your lipids and other risk factors
- Do NOT stop any medications that you think might be causing the problem without consulting with your doctor

Summary

Impotence is a treatable problem that is not the inevitable consequence of aging. Almost all patients with impotence can be treated. A thorough evaluation looking for the causes of impotence can be followed by the appropriate diagnostic testing, and then a multitude of treatment choices becomes available to assure that each patient has a successful outcome. In terms of determining which therapy is best for each individual, one must be informed of all the various possibilities, both about the cause of the impotence and the type of treatments that are available. None of the treatments will significantly affect the ability to have an orgasm. If needed, psychological support and counseling by a professional sexual counselor should be considered in many patients regardless of the cause of the impotence to help with any adjustments. **The first step is to have the courage to talk about it.**

Chapter 18

Improving Mental Health
and Lifestyle as We Age
Melodee Harris, MSN, APN

What is depression and what are the symptoms?
Depression is often described as a combination of symptoms such as sadness, anxiety, hopelessness or helplessness.

According to the American Psychiatric Association, a diagnosis of major depression is made when either depressed mood or loss of interest or pleasure occurs as one of five or more of the following symptoms listed below:

- Depressed mood
- Loss of interest in pleasurable activities
- Significant unintentional weight loss or weight gain
- Changes in sleep patterns
- Feelings of restlessness or feeling "slowed down"
- Fatigue or decreased energy
- Feelings of worthlessness or guilt
- Difficulty thinking, concentrating or making decisions
- Recurrent thoughts of death, suicide plans or attempts

Depressed mood or loss of pleasure must be present most of the day for more than two weeks and the symptoms must interfere with the ability of usual day-to-day functioning. A diagnosis of depression is not made if the symptoms can be explained by a physical condition.

What causes depression?
Sometimes I will hear older adults say, "My body and my mind just aren't what they used to be. Of course I am

depressed. I'm old." While there are a variety of factors that place the older adult at risk for depression, it is not natural or healthy to be depressed at any age. ***Old age is not the cause of depression.*** In fact, studies reveal that in general, older adults report feeling happier and more satisfied with life than younger populations.

Older adults are unique individuals with specific healthcare needs. So when symptoms of depression occur, it is a signal to seek help. ***No one should have to face depression alone.***

Older adults experience many physiological, age-related changes that can leave them at risk for depression. It is important to keep in mind that both physical and mental health are closely related. A slow response to physical or mental illness is a result of age-related changes. This slow response or decreased reserve capacity is due to such age-related changes as decreased lean muscle mass, decreased lung capacity, decreased kidney function, changes in hormones and immunity to disease. Slow response to a physical or mental illness can lead quickly to complications and serious illnesses.

Age-related changes that happen in the brain place older adults at risk for depression. Mood, personality and depression are regulated by specific areas of the brain that use substances known as ***neurotransmitters***. Neurotransmitters such as norepinephrine, serotonin and dopamine have an effect on symptoms of depression. Age-related changes that cause depression can be associated with chemical imbalances that occur by the way the brain produces and utilizes neurotransmitters. Physical illness and pain can also place stress upon the chemical balance in the brain. Sometimes depression may be seasonal or related to lack of exposure to sunlight that stimulates chemical release in the brain. It may take longer for older adults to respond to age-related

266

changes and produce the chemical balance needed to combat depression.

Who is at risk for depression?
History of Depression
Older adults with a history of depression are at risk for future episodes. Older adults may experience familiar symptoms that occurred in the past. Sometimes a family history of a close relative with depression can be a risk factor. However, late-life depression may occur in older adults who have not experienced any previous episodes.

Chronic illness or disability
Older adults who have multiple *chronic illnesses* such as diabetes, arthritis, cancer, kidney, lung or heart disease are also more likely to have depression. Often chronic illness is associated with *disability*. Illnesses such as diabetes occur simultaneously with other chronic illnesses. Managing multiple chronic illnesses on a day-to-day basis requires many resources for physical, mental, financial, and social support for the development of adequate *coping mechanisms*.

Depression is also very common in persons who have experienced sudden *disability* that occurs with motor vehicle accidents or other illnesses. This is partly due to the permanent physical limitation and disability that can occur. A lengthy rehabilitation on an inpatient or outpatient basis may be discouraging. Progress may be perceived as too slow and unrewarding without hope of a full recovery.

Depression is very common with *life-threatening illnesses* such as a heart attack. Sometimes after a heart attack or open-heart surgery, it takes time to gain back the confidence to perform physical activities. It may take longer for older adults to regain strength. Older adults may place unrealistic expectations upon the recovery phase from any life-threatening illness such as a heart attack or major surgery. The necessary *lifestyle changes* may seem to be an overwhelming task. Older adults may lose interest in activities that were once enjoyable and may experience a period of depression during this time of adjustment.

Neurological disorders such as stroke, Parkinson's disease or Alzheimer's disease place older adults at high risk for depression. Memory loss is caused by damage in the brain. This is a very frustrating experience for older adults. Another reason depression is so common in Parkinson's disease, dementia or among stroke patients is because of *chemical imbalances* due to damage in areas of the brain that control emotions. This can lead to embarrassment due to uncontrollable crying, laughing and depression. *Medication* can help restore chemical imbalances and relieve these symptoms.

Unmanaged pain
Untreated pain in persons with such diseases as cancer or arthritis can be a common cause of depression.

Social isolation
Not only can disease be limiting physically and functionally, but older adults also may tend to live in isolation because they find that activity associated with social interaction increases pain.

Side effects of medications
Medication side effects can play a role in depression. Certain prescription or over-the-counter medications can cause depression and *sexual dysfunction*. Many people are unaware of the side effects and interactions of medications or are reluctant to discuss these issues with health care

providers. All medications – including prescription, over-the-counter medications, herbs and vitamins – have possible side effects. It is important to discuss medication interactions and side effects with your healthcare provider and pharmacist.

Alcohol or substance abuse

Older adults with a history of *alcoholism* or *substance abuse* may experience a recurrence of *dependency* and are at high risk for depression. Alcoholism or substance abuse may be a way to self-medicate the symptoms of depression. Older adults who drink regular or excessive amounts of alcohol may minimize the problem or deny the abuse. Substituting alcohol for meals that results in *weight loss* is a cause of malnutrition. Early screening for depression and alcohol abuse by health care providers is very important.

Challenges associated with managing change as we age

Social and environmental changes may also contribute to depression. Perhaps more than any other phase of life, older age is a time of change. There may be declining health and changes in physical functioning. Sometimes older adults may experience *incontinence* or require *assistive devices* such as walkers or wheelchairs and are reluctant or embarrassed to venture out beyond a familiar environment. Many times there is not a *family member* or *financial means* for someone to help with physical activities. *Declining health* places older adults at high risk for depression. *Retirement* and other changes in lifestyle may precipitate depression. Retirement often leads to an identity crisis for older adults. Many older adults face retirement on a *fixed income*. Older age is also a time of *loss of loved ones*. Sometimes older adults may need to *downsize* and sell a home where they have lived most of their lives. If there is *too much change* or *change develops too rapidly*, older adults may feel a *loss of control* that can lead to depression.

269

Increase in stressful situations
The ability to manage stress is important at any age. Stress
that occurs with older age includes the stress from temporary
or chronic physical illness, family stress, stress associated
with employment and financial stress. Stress can result from
pleasurable experiences such as retirement, vacation and
marriage. The inability to deal with stress places older adults
at risk for depression.

Caregivers for loved ones
Older adults who are ***caregivers*** for a loved one are at high
risk for depression. Many older adults do not have the
financial means or other available help to meet the challenges
of care-giving. Being on-call 24 hours a day is an exhausting
task. Caregivers may feel exhausted, angry and isolated.
Many times caregivers will put off their own physical, mental
and social needs to care for a loved one. A substitute may
not be available to stay with a loved one so the caregiver can
schedule a doctor appointment or opportunities for regular
exercise. Church and social activities are often placed on
hold. There is also a significant financial burden. Caregivers
are often physically and mentally exhausted as well as
socially isolated, without anyone to share in support for the
burdens of caregiving, which leaves them at high risk for
depression.

How common is depression in the elderly?

Depression is very common in the geriatric population.
Often depression in the elderly remains undiagnosed and
untreated. There is a higher rate of suicide among adults
over 65 years old than in any other age group. While
depression is common among older adults, the notion that
most older adults are sick, depressed or in nursing homes is
not true. Only 5% of older adults live in a long-term care
facility. According to research studies and surveys, the

majority of older adults report feeling in good health and are happy with their lives.

How will I know if I am depressed?

Older adults have a *decreased reserve capacity to respond to physical illness*. For instance, an older adult with pneumonia may experience symptoms of *confusion* rather than an elevated temperature. An *elevated temperature* may be a late sign of a serious, life-threatening illness. *Sudden onset of confusion* with physical illness is referred to as *delirium*.

Just as older adults do not experience typical symptoms of physical disease, many times older adults do not experience typical symptoms of depression and may not feel sad. *Withdrawal from social activity* or the *inability to express emotion* also can indicate depression.

Sometimes family members or friends will be the first to realize something is wrong. *Changes in personality or mood* might be an indication of depression. Often *changes in physical appearance such as poor hygiene or grooming* will be one of the more obvious signs of depression. *Dependency upon alcohol, prescription medications or illicit drugs* is another indication of depression. *Preoccupation with thoughts of suicide* or *giving away possessions* may be nonverbal expressions of depression and intention of self-injury.

It is very important to distinguish between physical and mental causes of symptoms. *Many of the symptoms of physical illness are very similar to the symptoms of depression.* Fatigue, lack of energy and changes in appetite or sleep may indicate depression. However fatigue, lack of energy and appetite changes are also symptoms of a physical illness. This makes depression difficult to diagnose in older

271

adults. Delirium or symptoms that occur suddenly are more often the result of an acute physical illness that requires prompt attention. Misdiagnosis and delay in treatment for depression also interferes with recovery and quality of life.

What is the difference between memory loss and dementia?

Older adults with depression may experience some ***memory loss***. It is not uncommon for some memory loss to occur after a traumatic event or loss of a loved one. After treatment for depression or resolution of the crisis, full cognition is restored.

However, ***dementia*** is a progressive, terminal illness. Because of damage to areas of the brain that regulate mood and personality, depression is very common in persons with all types of dementia. It is likely that older adults with dementia will need treatment for depression at some stage of their illness. Dementia is irreversible and results in progressive neurological decline. Memory loss will not recover in persons with dementia.

What is the difference between bereavement/grief and depression?

Bereavement is different from depression. Bereavement is grief that occurs after loss of a loved one. ***Grief*** is categorized as a possible "expected" response to loss. While everyone is different, if feelings of sadness persist beyond two months or if the person is experiencing excessive guilt, worthlessness, inability to perform activities of daily living such as dressing, eating or personal hygiene, or hallucinations, the person may be depressed.

What should I do if I think I am depressed?

Sometimes older adults will say, "It's all in my head. I can handle this on my own. I do not need any help."

Take all symptoms of depression and thoughts of suicide, self-harm or harming others seriously.

It is important to seek help immediately by contacting your healthcare provider or going to the emergency room if you or a loved one experience any of the following symptoms of depression:

- Preoccupation with suicidal thoughts, self-injury or harming someone else
- Advanced depression
- Depression that is so severe it results in weight loss
- Delusional thoughts (thinking things that are not true such as everyone is out to get you) or hallucinations (seeing things that are not there)
- Alcohol or substance abuse

Often older adults may be reluctant to seek help because of negative social stigma associated with depression. Many times older adults may be afraid of the diagnosis. This may be because depression is often perceived as a personal weakness or a lack of self-control. This is not true. Depression is a physiological condition that requires treatment. While mild depression may pass with time, more advanced cases of depression require immediate treatment. Seeking professional help when symptoms develop can avoid a long course of recovery. Support from family loved ones or church members are as important in the diagnosis of depression as in any physical illness. There are many community support groups that may also be helpful.

Recognizing that something is wrong is the first step in feeling better. If you feel depressed, seek help from your healthcare provider. Like any other change in health status, early diagnosis and treatment is important. Seeking

273

treatment for depression is especially important to older adults for maintaining function and independence.

Because depression is a very treatable illness on an outpatient basis, your primary healthcare provider will be able to diagnose and treat symptoms of depression. Patient rights have come a long way. In addition, conditions like depression are better understood and can be treated and monitored effectively by knowledgeable health care providers. Should a referral to a psychiatrist or hospitalization become necessary, healthcare providers and office staff are trained to comply with federal requirements to keep patient confidentiality.

Why is it so important for older adults to seek treatment for depression?

Treating depression is important at any age. Depression affects sleeping, eating and the ability to function in day-to-day activities that are important to the independence of older adults. The inability to function on a day-to-day basis can lead to hospitalization or nursing home placement. In addition, seeking help early in the course of any condition is the key to prevention of serious complications and shorter recovery time.

What is the treatment for depression?

It is important to find a healthcare provider you trust. This is important in the treatment of any condition. Your health care provider will ask questions about eating, sleeping, sexual activity, social activities and how you are feeling emotionally. Answering the questions honestly will help treatment decisions. You may find it embarrassing or uncomfortable to discuss your private life. This is normal. However, expressing feelings to a healthcare provider you trust may also be a relief.

Because appetite changes are often symptoms of depression, your healthcare provider may recommend ways to improve appetite and eat regular meals. Sleep patterns may also be discussed. A healthy diet and adequate rest have many physical and mental health benefits.

Becoming more involved in social or church activities may be another topic for discussion. Your healthcare provider may also recommend psychotherapy with a qualified therapist.

While there are many non-pharmacological approaches to the treatment of depression, medication may also be prescribed.

What types of medications will be prescribed?

Antidepressants are prescribed for depression. There are many new classifications of antidepressants that are safer and more effective in older adults than older medications. There are many areas of the brain that provide neurological pathways for regulating symptoms of depression through medication. This is the reason there are several classifications of antidepressants.

Serotonin reuptake inhibitors (often referred to as *SSRI's*) are one class of the newer, most commonly prescribed medications for older adults. Depression can occur with a lack of serotonin, a neurotransmitter in the brain. These medications can make more serotonin available and decrease symptoms of depression. Other classifications of prescription drugs treat areas of the brain that may be affected by neurotransmitter imbalance.

Medications that stimulate appetite or help with sleep may be prescribed. *Antipsychotics* may be prescribed to help control delusions or hallucinations sometimes associated with depression.

What are the side effects of antidepressants?

Side effects can vary depending upon the drug classification. However, common side effects of antidepressants can be dizziness, light-headedness, change in blood pressure, sleepiness, or falls. ***Remember that all herbal, over-the-counter or prescription medications have possible side effects.*** Antidepressants can interact with over-the-counter or prescription medications you may be taking for other conditions. ***Alcohol and certain foods may also interact with some antidepressants.***

Keep in mind that everyone is different. Older adults may require a decreased dose of a prescribed antidepressant. It takes communication between you and your doctor to help determine the dosage that will be effective to treat your depression. It is important to discuss the side effects of antidepressants with your healthcare provider and pharmacist.

How should I take my medications?

Always follow your doctor's instructions for taking medications. ***Talk with your doctor about all the medication you are taking***, including prescription, herbal and over-the-counter medications. It is helpful to bring all your medications with you in the original bottles so your doctor can evaluate the medications and how you are taking them. It is also very helpful to obtain your medications from one pharmacy. Multiple healthcare providers and multiple pharmacies can be a significant barrier to determining the effectiveness of medications and side effects.

It may take several weeks to more than a month to notice a difference in symptoms of depression. While it is important to prescribe only the necessary medication to reduce side effects and cost, sometimes more than one antidepressant will be prescribed. A partial response to an antidepressant may mean that more than one area of the brain could be responsible for your symptoms. Since there is not one medication that works on every aspect of the brain involved in the symptoms of depression, additional medication may be required. It is important to communicate with your health care provider and keep follow-up appointments to monitor your progress.

Antidepressants are different from taking a pain pill that can provide immediate relief. Antidepressants work more gradually. This is why you will need to work closely with your healthcare provider and avoid self-medicating by starting or stopping the medication on your own.

While the exact time may vary, it may take a trial of about one year to avoid a relapse of depression before discontinuing the antidepressant. If an antidepressant is discontinued too soon and a relapse of depression is experienced, a longer trial may be necessary.

Talk with your health care provider about trying over-the-counter medications and herbal remedies. Alternative therapies have side effects that can interfere with other medications. While alternative medication therapy may be less expensive, often safety has not been established. Medications that meet FDA approval are tested for effectiveness, documentation of side effects and dosage needed to produce the desired outcome.

What can I do to treat depression without taking medication?

While medication may be necessary, three simple ways to prevent depression can be summed up in a quote attributed to Tom Bodett, *"They say a person needs just three things to*

277

be happy in this world: Someone to love, something to do and something to hope for."

From the moment we enter this world to the end of life, having someone to love is important to human beings. Older adults who experience the loss of a spouse, family and loss of friends know how important it is to have someone to love. Someone to love may be a member of your family, church group or friends. Pets can also be very important companions. It is not too late to fall in love with someone who has similar interests and desires for sharing life experiences.

Something to do and a purpose in life can prevent depression. Something to do can improve responses to pain and help older adults stay engaged and active. In fact, many older adults continue to enjoy careers late in life, take on a second career or volunteer work. Retirement is also described by many older adults as a time of new and exciting opportunities to enjoy life.

For many older adults, something to hope for is often found in spiritual experiences and faith. Spirituality provides comfort for physical and emotional pain. A positive attitude is an important strategy for prevention of depression in older adults.

What are the lifestyle changes I will need to make to prevent depression?

Prevention and education are the keys to optimal physical and mental health. The most important health promotion and prevention concerns for older adults are maintenance of functioning and quality of life. Depression can lead to alterations in activities of daily living and rob older adults of independence. An awareness of the symptoms of depression nd the negative outcomes associated with depression is a good place to start.

Because changes in appetite can be one of the symptoms of depression, *it is important for older adults to be aware of overeating or lack of appetite*. While depression can cause overeating that predisposes the older adult to illnesses such as diabetes, high blood pressure or heart disease; lack of appetite is associated with more negative outcomes for older adults.

Age-related changes in the hypothalamus of the brain often prevent older adults from recognizing hunger or thirst. Other age-related changes diminish the reserve capacity or the ability to fight off disease. Electrolyte imbalances, decreased immunity or other consequences of malnutrition or dehydration make the health status of the older adult especially vulnerable.

Disturbed sleep is also a symptom of depression. Persons with depression may notice sleep patterns that include a longer time in bed with early arousals spent in worry and anxiety. Establishing a nightly routine, turning off the television, prayer, listening to comforting music are all ways to avoid sleep deprivation that are associated with feelings of depression. *Exposure to natural sunlight* may improve disturbed sleep as well as symptoms of depression. Many research studies report that older adults who *engage in regular physical exercise* find they not only benefit physically, but are happier and have a better quality of life than older adults who are more sedentary. Our brains release endorphins during exercise that can help prevent depression.

Engaging in social, community or church activities is very important in the prevention of depression for older adults. *Staying active and making new friends is very important to successful aging.* Older adults may help elementary children in reading programs or serve as surrogate grandparents. There are many opportunities for older adults to make a difference in the community.

If you are an older adult with depression, see your healthcare provider. Take the first steps toward help and hope for a healthier tomorrow by living life to its fullest today!

Chapter 19

Common Orthopedic Problems Encountered as We Age

Michael Pyevich, MD, Timothy Milea, MD,
Joseph G. Martin, MD, Steven A. Boardman, MD, and
Richard S. Collins, MD

As we get older, we often find that our bones ache and we experience orthopedic problems. Some of the more common challenges are discussed below.

My shoulder hurts especially at night and when reaching behind my back. Is this just "old age" and arthritis?

Episodes of *shoulder pain* are very common in many age groups but only occasionally are they caused by "*arthritis*." *Arthritis of the shoulder* refers to inflammation around the shoulder because the normally smooth cartilage surfaces of the shoulder joint are worn and rough. This can be caused by previous trauma, rheumatologic diseases, and even infection. However, in most cases, no cause is readily identifiable.

The treatment of arthritis of the shoulder is based not on a patient's X-rays but on the severity of the patient's symptoms. The common treatments include *activity modification*, *nonsteroidal anti-inflammatory medications*, and occasional *injections of corticosteroid medication*. Pain associated with arthritis of the shoulder may even require *shoulder replacement*.

While arthritic conditions of the shoulder certainly do occur and can cause significant pain, conditions of the *rotator cuff* (a tendinous structure within the shoulder) are a much more common cause of *shoulder pain*. Muscles from around the *shoulder blade* (*scapula*) come together and form a sleeve-shaped tendon called the ***rotator cuff***. The rotator cuff reaches out from the scapula to the head of the ***humerus*** and helps to hold the head of the humerus within the socket (***glenoid***) of the scapula. It also helps to provide and coordinate rotational movement of the arm. In many shoulders, the rotator cuff experiences age-related degeneration and consequent dysfunction, which allows discoordinated movement of the shoulder joint during rotation. This allows ***impingement*** (bumping and scuffing) of the rotator cuff on surrounding areas of bone and subsequent ***tendonitis*** of the rotator cuff. This may resolve with time and may also be helped with physical therapy and occasionally a corticosteroid injection. In some cases this does not resolve and an ***arthroscopic procedure*** to remove a small amount of surrounding bone may help to allow the tendonitis to resolve.

In some patients the rotator cuff impinges to the point that it may tear within itself or from its attachment on the head of the humerus. This is called a ***rotator cuff tear*** and may successfully be treated with physical therapy and corticosteroid injections. However, many times it may require surgical repair of the rotator cuff followed by extensive physical therapy.

Finally, in some patients the rotator cuff may tear so completely that it may not be repairable and may then cause a severely arthritic condition of the shoulder. This most severe form of rotator cuff disease may be treated once again with physical therapy and corticosteroid injections. However, if this is not successful and the pain in shoulder is severe, then a specially designed ***shoulder replacement*** called ***reverse shoulder arthroplasty*** can be performed and achieve excellent pain relief and function in many patients.

Finally, though modern imaging such as X-rays and MRI

elped to diagnose conditions of the shoulder, they do not dictate treatment. The severity of the patient's symptoms dictates the treatment, not the X-rays.

'm having trouble with my knee. Should I get a knee replacement?

The main reason to get a joint replacement is for pain relief from arthritis. Most people who have knee replacement surgery are having difficulty walking significant distances because of pain. This can interfere with work and recreational activities. Some people require a cane to walk, though cane use is less common than it used to be. Difficulty climbing stairs is also a common complaint. People who need a knee replacement frequently have pain in their knee even while resting, and sometimes have difficulty with sleep because of it.

People who need a knee replacement will have significant signs of wear and tear shown on their knee X-ray. Your doctor should be suspicious of other causes of pain if your X-ray is normal. Typically, your doctor will recommend that you try medicine for your arthritis pain, and sometimes injections are suggested. When these are no longer adequate, surgery may be necessary.

There is no set age for joint replacement. People in their 90's have knee replacements if they are healthy enough to tolerate the surgery. Younger patients are encouraged to wait as long as possible before having knee replacement. This is because the older you are when you have it, the more likely it is that it will last the rest of your life. It is not a good idea, though, to wait so long that inactivity becomes the cause of other health problems.

Be sure to learn about knee replacement surgery. People

frequently seek advice from people who have already had the surgery. The Internet can be a source of information, but you must be careful not to accept all the information you find at face value. Of course, your physician is probably your best resource. Knee replacement has helped many people feel better and be more active. It may be that it could help you too.

I've been having knee pain and my family doctor told me I should see an orthopedic surgeon. What exactly is an orthopedic surgeon and when do I really need to see one?

An *orthopedic surgeon* is a medical doctor that specializes in disorders of the musculoskeletal system, that is, problems with bones, joints, and muscles. An orthopedic surgeon went to medical school and then spent at least 5 additional years concentrating on all aspects of orthopedics. An orthopedic surgeon treats broken bones, arthritis, sports injuries, tendonitis, bursitis, disorders of the spine, deformities from birth and countless other issues relating to aches and pains of the body. A rheumatologist treats some of the same things, but an orthopedist is extensively trained in the surgical intervention of these disorders, in addition to the non-surgical treatment options.

Your family doctor may very well start some form of treatment for your ailment at the outset, but if you fail to improve over a few weeks time, your doctor will often opt to refer you to an orthopedic surgeon to further evaluate your problem. Your evaluation will usually involve telling the orthopedist the details of your injury (if there was one), your symptoms, what you've tried in the past to help the symptoms, a physical examination concentrated on the ailing body part (and all associated bones and joints) and an X-ray examination. This may be enough to determine the diagnosis and institute a treatment regimen. However, sometimes additional testing may be needed, such as an MRI, a CT scan, blood work or some other tests.

Most problems ultimately can be treated without surgery, but some require surgical treatment. You and your orthopedist will together come up with the appropriate treatment for you and your ailment.

My doctor told me that I need a total knee replacement. Are there any other options for knee arthritis?

Before considering a *total knee replacement*, the orthopedist usually tries other non-operative methods of treatment, such as an exercise program and medication. An exercise program can strengthen the muscles around the knee joint and medications can decrease the inflammation in the arthritic knee. The most common medications used are *nonsteroidal anti-inflammatory drugs*, or *NSAIDs*. Commonly prescribed NSAIDs are *ibuprofen* and *naproxen*, but there are several others.

Additional non-operative treatments for knee arthritis include injecting the knee with either a corticosteroid or one of the viscosupplementation agents, using a cane or a crutch or recommending a brace. 40% of body weight can be unloaded by using a cane or a crutch, which can reduce pain. Some patients do not like the stigma of using a cane, however, and therefore opt not to use one. An injection into the knee with corticosterioid (cortisone) can reduce the inflammation in the joint, but the results can be somewhat unpredictable. It may work well initially, but may not give long-standing relief. The *viscosupplements* (made from rooster combs) have also met with success in the right patient. Their exact mode of action is not really known, but has been shown to work at least as well as the NSAIDs. Braces can unload the inner or outer arthritic aspect of the knee to relieve pain, but can be cumbersome.

There are surgical options other than total knee replacement that can be performed in the right patient. If the arthritis is not severe on X-ray, it may be possible to put a small camera in the joint (arthroscopy) and smooth down rough cartilage and remove any tears in the cartilage of the knee. Another possibility may be to change the alignment of the knee by tipping the shin bone into different alignment to unload the arthritic part of the knee. Finally, there is a knee replacement available that only replaces the arthritic "part" of the knee as opposed to a "total" knee replacement. This is called a ***unicompartmental knee replacement***, which leaves much more of the patient's normal bone and cartilage intact. This

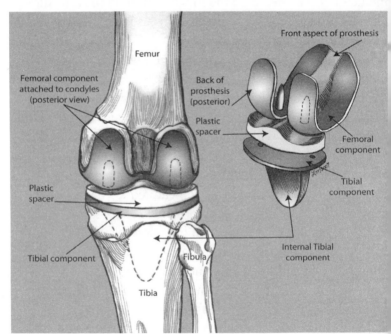

Figure 1. Knee prosthesis (posterior view)

can be a good option in the right patient.

None of these options is ideal for everyone. Total knee replacement may, in fact, be the best option in some cases. You and your orthopedist should discuss all options and decide which is best for your situation.

I'm 58 years old and I like to jog but my wife tells me that I'm too old and that I'm doing damage to my joints. Is this true?

There is no doubt that exercise is beneficial in multiple ways throughout our lives. And as we get older, continuing to exercise produces continued health benefits including lowering the risk for coronary disease and diabetes, combating obesity and osteoporosis, maintaining muscular strength and endurance, and there's even evidence that exercise can protect the aging brain from dementia and Alzheimer's disease.

For those individuals that have led a relatively sedentary life style and wish to begin an exercise regimen, ***overuse injuries*** are the most common challenges older athletes face. The incidence of exertion-related cardiovascular events is also greater among older athletes, especially men, and therefore medical status is imperative to know prior to starting a new exercise program. Age is not a limiting factor to exercising, but a more gradual approach in implementing an exercise program at older ages seems most prudent. In addition, many health benefits from physical activity can be achieved at lower intensities.

The type of exercise chosen is dependent on the individual. For someone that has been exercising for many years, there is no reason he or she can't continue that same exercise indefinitely. However, injuries sustained during childhood and adolescence may compromise function in later life, limiting the type of activity. In addition, even in the absence of injury, vigorous participation in sports and fitness activities during childhood and adolescence has been shown to possibly increase the likelihood of developing *osteoarthritis*, yet little effort has been made to document long-term consequences of continued sports participation. For those individuals that have arthritic knees, hips, or ankles, low-impact exercise is clearly a better choice of exercise than high impact activities. Examples of *low-impact activities* are walking, swimming, biking, golf and elliptical machines. Examples of *high-impact activities* are jogging, racquetball, and basketball. That being said, however, there is no hard evidence that shows running or jogging later in life is any harder on our joints than at any other time.

It's my understanding that breaking a hip is common. What do I need to know about breaking a hip?

Hip fractures are very common. Due to the increasing elderly population, the estimated number of hip fractures worldwide will rise from 1.7 million in 1990 to 6.3 million in 2050. This estimate assumes a stable rate of hip fractures. But if the hip fracture rate rises by just 1%, the number of hip fractures worldwide could be as high as 8.2 million by 2050.

The hip is a "ball and socket" joint where the round ball of the upper thigh bone fits into the bowl-shaped socket (the *acetabulum*) of the pelvis. A "hip fracture" means a person broke the upper part of the thighbone, near where the thighbone fits into the hip joint. It does not mean a fracture of the pelvis. Fractures of the pelvis and acetabulum do occur, but they are not as common, nor are they called hip fractures.

Most hip fractures happen to people who are 65 or older. Falls cause most hip fractures, so if you are in this age group, you need to be extra careful to avoid falls, even minor falls. This is in contrast to children and young adults, in whom hip fractures are very rare, and when they do occur, usually are due to a high-energy trauma (e.g., car accident).

As we get older, our bones naturally lose some strength and are more likely to break, even from a minor fall.

Hip fractures are most common in older women. This is true for several reasons. Men naturally have stronger bones than women. And when women go through menopause, they lose estrogen. This makes it more likely that they will develop *osteoporosis*, a disease that causes bones to thin. Osteoporosis greatly increases the risk of a hip fracture. Osteoporosis is discussed in much greater detail in other areas of this book.

A hip fracture is more than a broken bone. If you are older, breaking your hip can mean a major change in your life. You will likely need surgery, and it can take as long as a year to recover. It is possible to get back to very near normal with time, physical therapy, perseverance, and support; however, some older people never will get back to their pre-injury level of activity and may not be able to live independently once they do recover. After your surgery, it will be hard for you to do things yourself. You will need to go to a nursing home or rehabilitation center for a while after your surgery. But the more active you can be in your care, the faster you will get better.

Finally, prevent a hip fracture if possible. Preventing osteoporosis is extremely important and is discussed in detail in other parts of this book. In addition, move loose throw rugs and move any extension cords. Get any trip hazards up and out of your way. Always turn a light on and put your glasses on when moving about your house at night. Wear sturdy, flat-soled shoes. Put grab bars up in your bathroom. In this case, an ounce of prevention is truly worth a pound of cure.

My 78-year-old wife broke her hip and the orthopedic surgeon says he needs to surgically replace part of her bone with metal. Can't she just let it heal on its own, and if not, then why can't he simply fix the broken bone and not replace it?

There are two types of hip fractures: a *femoral neck fracture* and an *intertrochanteric hip fracture*. Both involve breaking the upper part of their thighbone, near where the thighbone fits into the hip joint, but they are treated differently. Almost 100% of the time, the treatment of choice that will give the best outcome for any patient of any age will be surgical treatment for both of these hip fractures.

Surgery is the most prudent thing to do in most cases. With surgery, your wife can start getting out of bed the very next day (with the help of the physical therapists). If your wife's hip fracture were treated without surgery, she would have to lie in bed for at least 8 weeks, and in that time frame, an elderly person becomes quite debilitated, can get bed sores, risks potentially fatal conditions such as lung problems and blood clots, loses tremendous amounts of strength, muscle mass, and endurance, and has chronic pain in the hip with any attempt at moving (such as sponge bathing or getting on/off a bedpan) because the broken ends of the bone move against each other until it starts to heal. Realistically, elderly patients that have their hip fractures treated without surgery will usually never walk again.

Maintaining strength and endurance is hard enough after

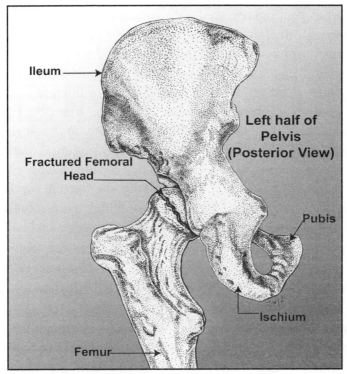

Figure 2. Fractured Femoral Head

surgery, but we can get the patient moving immediately after surgery to prevent the rapid decline in lung function, prevent blood clots and prevent the rapid decline in strength. In addition, once the pain from the incision is gone, surgically treated patients are much more comfortable because their fracture is now stabilized. Surgery usually works well, but you will need to be patient. Getting better can take a long time, and you may never be able to get around as well as you could before.

That being said, then, the type of surgery you have will depend on where the break is and how bad it is. Your doctor may put metal screws, pins, a rod, or a plate and screws in your hip to fix the break. Or you may need to have all or part of your hip replaced. Regarding the femoral neck fractures, if the fracture is still in excellent alignment, then the blood supply to the ball is still okay, and it can be treated quite simply with some screws placed through a one-inch incision. However, it sounds like the type of fracture your wife has is a displaced femoral neck fracture, where the ball is knocked off the end of the thighbone and is no longer in good alignment. The problem with simply putting the ball back on and fixing it with screws is that the blood supply to the ball has been lost. The ball will die, the fracture won't heal, and she'd need a hip replacement within a few months. But by replacing the ball of her thighbone with a metal ball, these issues are resolved.

I need a hip replacement. Is the minimally-invasive hip replacement best for me?

Hip replacement is a very common surgical treatment for pain from severe hip arthritis that is not responsive to non-surgical treatments. Once the decision has been made to proceed with hip replacement, your orthopedic surgeon will discuss the surgical approach with you. The standard hip replacement leaves a scar somewhere around 8 inches, depending on the size of the patient and the approach used by the surgeon. The minimally-invasive and 2-incision approaches can leave smaller scars, and less cutting sounds like a good thing. But knowing the right questions to ask is a key to determining if this new technique is for you.

Theoretical advantages of minimally-invasive hip replacement are less blood loss, less post-operative pain, decreased hospital stays, improved scar appearance and quicker healing. In the hands of properly trained surgeons, proponents state that patients can expect benefits that are vastly improved; that patients can even go home the same day as surgery and can walk without crutches within a week.

roponents state the quicker recovery is because the surgical
chnique splits muscles and tendons rather than cutting
em.

urrent research, however, shows that patients often fare
o better with minimally-invasive hip replacement than
ose having a standard hip replacement – and may, in fact,
o worse. Critics say benefits of minimally-invasive hip
eplacement are still unproven and that the smaller incision
acrifices the surgeon's visualization, which can lead to
oor positioning of hip implants occuring more frequently.
his, in turn, can lead to hip dislocations or failure in the
onger term. This is true even in very experienced surgeons.
ne study indicated that even when the less-invasive
echnique was performed by a very experienced surgeon, the
omplication rate was nearly four times higher than normal,
nd the complications were also more serious.

inally, the minimally-invasive techniques are not for every
atient. One can think of it like this: A surgical incision fits
 patient like a dress fits a patient – some patients are a size 4,
ome are a size 16.

Minimally-invasive techniques are still being studied and the
echniques perfected. The minimally-invasive technique may
e the right choice for you. Discuss it in detail with your
urgeon.

**broke my wrist years ago, and my husband
ust fractured his wrist. What's the difference
etween a bone that's broken and one that is
ractured?**

ou say "tomato," I say . . . They mean the same thing. A
one that is broken is also fractured, cracked, busted, etc.
"*Fracture*" simply sounds more like a medical term. It's

like saying "epistaxis" instead of "nose bleed." They mean the same thing.

The dictionary's definition of the verb "fracture" is "to break." From a bone's perspective, a fracture in a bone means that the integrity of the bone has been lost or damaged; that is, it's been broken.

There are many types of fractures, however, and many ways to describe how severe a fracture is. First of all, every single bone in your body, from the top of your head (cranium cerebrale) to your toes (phalanges), can be broken or fractured. Second, we want to know if the fracture is *displaced* (the bone edges that are broken are not well-approximated) or not. We want to know if the fractured bone is in good alignment or *angulated*. We want to know if the fracture in the bone is straight across (*transverse*), angled (*oblique*) or very long and oblique (*spiral*). We want to know if the fracture is in many little pieces (*comminuted*) or in two main pieces (*simple*). Formerly, when people used to talk about a "clean break," they were talking about a simple, non-displaced fracture. We don't use this term any longer. Finally we want to know if the break in the bone is in the middle of the bone (*diaphyseal*), the end of the bone (*metaphyseal*), or into the joint (*intra-articular*). All of these characteristics of the fracture help us in determining the best way to treat the fracture.

Some special considerations about fractures we also need to know are, for example, if the fracture is in a child, we want to know if the fracture involves the growth plate. In a high-energy trauma, we need to know if the fracture is open (the bone is sticking out of the skin) or closed (the skin's integrity is still intact). Formerly, when people used to talk about "compound fractures," they were talking about whether or not the bone was out of the skin (compound) or not. We

294

on't use this term any longer. If the fracture occurs through tumor (whether it be a benign or a malignant tumor) in the bone or any area of bone that has been weakened by a disease process, we call this a *"pathologic fracture."* The osteoporosis-related fractures of the hip, spine and wrist in the elderly used to be included in the group of pathologic fractures. And they truly are because the bone has been weakened and is not normal. But with our increasing awareness of the osteoporosis epidemic, we have given this type of fracture its own name: *"Fragility fractures,"* because the bone is indeed fragile.

My foot is flat and seems to be getting worse with age. It is now bothering me quite a bit. Can this be fixed?

Flatfoot is frequently encountered in the adult population. Adult flatfoot is a foot condition characterized by partial or complete loss (collapse) of *the medial longitudinal arch*.

The adult flatfoot is often a complex disorder with a diversity of symptoms and various degrees of deformity. In many adults, a *low arch* or a flatfoot is painless and causes no problems.

However, a painful flatfoot can be a sign of a congenital abnormality or an injury to the muscles and tendons of the foot. Flat feet can even contribute to low back pain. If the condition progresses, you may experience problems with walking, climbing stairs and wearing shoes. Your feet may tire easily or become painful with prolonged standing. It may be difficult to move your heel or midfoot around, or to stand on your toes. Your foot may ache, particularly in the heel or arch area, with swelling along the inner side. Pain symptoms are caused by changes along the inner foot and *plantar arch*, as well as by collapse through the *midfoot*

295

and impingement along the outer aspect of the *hindfoot*.
The *ankle bone* (*talus*) does not align normally with the
heel bone (*calcaneus*), or the small bones of the midfoot.
Muscles in the leg and foot tend to fatigue and cramp because
of overuse.

It's been estimated that 5 to 10% of the adult population
is flatfooted. But it's usually the stiff, rigid, non-flexible
adult flatfoot that is most symptomatic. The deformity may
be associated with pain, instability and severe functional
limitations or it may be of little clinical significance.
Associated conditions such as rheumatoid arthritis or diabetes
may be significant in the patient with adult flatfoot (about
half of all people with rheumatoid arthritis will develop a
progressive flatfoot deformity). Occupation, activity level,
obesity, footwear and history of trauma also play a role.

There's an easy way to tell if you have flat feet. Simply wet
your feet, then stand on a flat, dry surface that will leave an
imprint of your foot. A normal footprint has a wide band
connecting the ball of the foot to the heel, with an indentation
on the inner side of the foot. A foot with a high arch has a
large indentation and a very narrow connecting band. Flat
feet leave a nearly complete imprint, with almost no inward
curve where the arch should be.

Most people have "*flexible flatfoot*" as children; an arch is
visible when the child rises up on the toes, but not when the
child is standing. As you age, the tendons that attach to the
bones of the foot grow stronger and tighten, forming the
arch. But if injury damages the tendons, the arch can "fall,"
creating a flatfoot.

Although you can do the "wet test" at home, a thorough
examination by an orthopedist will be needed to identify why

he flatfoot developed. Possible causes include a congenital abnormality, a bone fracture or dislocation, a torn or stretched tendon, arthritis or neurologic weakness.

What types of treatment are available for flatfoot?

A painless flatfoot that does not hinder your ability to walk or wear shoes requires no particular treatment. But for the painful flatfoot, treatment options depend on the cause and shape of the foot. Non-surgical treatment options include: making shoe modifications, using custom-made orthotic devices/arch supports, nonsteroidal anti-inflammatory medications, braces and physical therapy.

In some cases, surgery may be needed to correct the problem. Surgical options include: *arthrodesis*, or fusing, one or more of the bones in the foot/ankle together; *osteotomy*, or cutting a bone to correct alignment; or *tendon reconstruction*.

Recovery from a surgery often requires 6-8 weeks of not putting weight on the foot and up to 3 months in a cast. So it's not a simple recovery by any means, but the outcome is usually very favorable.

I have had a bunion for years, and it seems to be getting worse. What causes this?

Bunions are a common problem manifested as a bony bump on the inner aspect of the big toe (the bunion) and the big toe angled towards the other toes (*hallux valgus*). These can hurt or they may be completely pain-free. Pain from bunions is often mechanical, meaning the pain comes from direct pressure of a shoe over the bump or from the malalignment of the big toe joint. There are also conditions that people think are "bunions" and they're not, such as a bad case of arthritis (a condition called ***hallux rigidus***) at the big toe joint. Your orthopedist can tell you exactly what condition you have.

There is some discrepancy as to what causes bunions. Depending on what article you read, you'll get varying opinions. You'll read that bunions are caused 100% from improper or unsuitable footwear. You'll also read that genetic predisposition (heredity) is the predominant causative factor for bunions. The fact of the matter is that both opinions are correct. It's a mixture of the two that causes bunions.

Improper footwear is felt to be fashionable shoes with high heels and small, narrow, pointy toe boxes that cram the toes all together. It's the type of shoe my wife calls "cute." Just to show that these types of shoes play a role, consider these facts:

Bunions are much more common in females. The higher frequency in females may be related to the strong link between footwear fashion and bunions.

Second, bunions occur in about 3% of the population in countries where people wear non-Western style shoes. They occur in about 33% of the population in Western countries.

Third, nearly 90% of women wear dress shoes that are at least one size too small or too narrow, and others have reported that the average woman in the U.S. wears a dress shoe up to 2-1/2 sizes too small.

Finally, women's feet change shape as they age, whether or not they get bunions. A woman should get rid of shoes that are at least 10 years old, because her foot has changed shape over time to the point where the older shoes do not actually fit any more.

So, shoes certainly play a role, but that's not the entire story. Patients who develop bunions often seem to also have a genetic tendency to do so. As stated earlier, even in countries without Western-style shoes, about 3% of the population will develop a bunion.

A strong family history of bunions can increase the likelihood of developing this foot disorder. After all, there are men that get bunions that don't wear high heels. And some adolescent girls get bunions before they get the chance to wear improper footwear.

We don't know why bunions occur in these instances, we can simply explain it away as "genetics."

We do know that various other conditions, such as arthritis and several genetic and neuromuscular diseases, can cause muscle imbalances and resultant bunions, but this is relatively rare in the general population.

However, once a bunion has formed, the mechanics of the feet and toes are altered. Tendons begin to pull the toe into an abnormal position, and the problem may worsen over time. A hammertoe of the second toe can occur as the big toe slides under the second toe. However, that is not a certain fate; some bunions/hallux valgus get worse to a point and then don't worsen. Time will tell, but try to avoid those fashionable shoes.

My bunions hurt. What can I do?

Pain from a bunion is usually mechanical, that is, from direct pressure of a shoe over the bump or from the malalignment of the big toe joint. The abnormal big toe joint can get inflamed and hurt. As the inflammation worsens, people can experience pain with shoe wear and walking. Finally, if a bunion is bad enough and a hammertoe develops in the 2nd toe, this can be a source of pain either on top of the stiff 2nd toe or in the ball of the foot under the 2nd toe. Your orthopedist will also let you know if you have a bad case of arthritis at the big toe joint (hallux rigidus), because this can also cause pain, and some of the treatments for hallux rigidus are the same as for hallux valgus (bunions).

Treatment of bunions is usually conservative at first and usually means wearing more appropriate footwear. This does not necessarily imply wearing bulky orthopedic shoes, but it does require that you find comfortable shoes with a wider toe box. Shoes can also be stretched in the toebox to make more room for the bump of the bunion. If your symptoms are only present when wearing shoes, changing or stretching your shoes may be all you have to do. That's the good news.

The bad news is that if modifying your footwear doesn't relieve your symptoms, then the decision has to be made between a) living with it, or b) having surgery. There is no other non-surgical treatment for a bunion. Many things have been tried in the past. There have been all sorts of straps and spacers and splints and contraptions that you'd wear either in your shoe or at night while sleeping, and none of these has ever made a difference.

If surgery is contemplated, it must be done for the right reason: pain. There is no other reason to perform surgery on a bunion. The World's Biggest and Ugliest Bunion, if pain-free, should not be treated with surgery. If it ever becomes painful and shoe changes don't make a difference, then do surgery. Feet are for function, not appearance. There are women who like to wear sandals and paint their nails that would disagree with me, but I will not operate on a bunion that does not hurt. I am not making a personal statement against cosmetic surgery. I have no problems with facelifts

300

or nose jobs. But we don't walk on our faces or noses. We walk on our feet and no truer statement has ever been said: "You take your feet for granted until they hurt." There are too many potential complications to perform a bunion surgery simply for cosmetic reasons. While improved cosmesis is an effect of surgical treatment, the procedure should be done because of pain and difficulty with footwear. The goal of surgery is to relieve pain and restore normal mechanics to the foot, and patients must have realistic expectations.

Rarely, the bunion can simply be shaved off, but usually the surgical treatment of a bunion is more extensive — otherwise the bunion will simply return over time. Bunion surgery involves breaking one or more bones to correct the alignment, and tendon/ligament reconstructions, so the toe points in the proper direction. The major drawback to bunion surgery is that you will have pain in the foot, swelling for 6 months or so, and probably will not be completely healed for about nine months. The most common complication of bunion surgery is a recurrence of the bunion months or years later. Other potential complications of surgery include inadequate correction, overcorrection of the deformity (hallux varus — the big toe points inward), nerve injury, infection and the bone not healing. Depending on the type of surgery you have, you may be able to walk on the foot right away, or you may be on crutches for 6 weeks. The patients who tend to be dissatisfied with bunion surgery are those patients who are having surgery done to allow them to have normal-looking feet or allow them to wear slim shoes. As mentioned, this is a mistake.

When I stand or walk for more than a few minutes, my back and legs start to ache, get numb and tingle, and feel weak. Then, when I sit down or lean forward, they get better.

There are many reasons that people can experience symptoms of pain, weakness, and sensation changes in the legs. These include blood supply problems, nerve function changes due to diabetes, and some arthritic problems in the hips and knees. However, a very common problem that is associated with aging of the lumbar spine is *spinal stenosis*.

Spinal stenosis is the term used to describe narrowing of the canal in the spine through which the nerves travel. A few cases occur due to a narrow canal from birth, but the vast majority are a result of degenerative and arthritic changes that occur over many years. It most commonly occurs in people over 50 years of age. Normal wear-and-tear occurs in the spine in all of us over time, and spinal stenosis can occur in anyone, regardless of the type of work or recreational activities in the individual's lifetime.

As the spine ages, several changes occur. The ligaments that help support the spine thicken as a result of calcium deposits. The small joints of the spine become arthritic and enlarge with bone spurs. Discs between the vertebrae of the spine narrow and can thicken or bulge into the nerve canal. All of these factors combine to cause narrowing of the nerve canal, and can then lead to symptoms of spinal stenosis. Less commonly, the arthritic changes can lead to some instability of the vertebrae, leading to slippage of one vertebra on another.

What types of treatment are available for spinal stenosis?

Many treatments are available for symptoms of spinal

stenosis. As with most problems, the simplest treatments are used first. Anti-inflammatory medications, either over-the-counter or prescription, can be tried. Physical therapy is often effective to help improve the strength and flexibility of the arthritic spine. Spinal injections (epidural injections) are often used for cases that are not responsive to simpler treatments.

Surgical treatment is used in cases when non-surgical measures have not provided adequate control of the symptoms. The most common operation is called a ***decompressive laminectomy***. The lamina is the covering of bone on the back of each vertebra that covers the nerve canal. When the lamina is removed, the canal size increases, and the surgeon can then remove the bone spurs and thickened ligaments that are compressing the nerves. In cases where there is some instability of the spine, a fusion may be recommended. This usually includes the use of screws and rods to help the vertebrae fuse together.

A more recent addition to surgical treatment for spinal stenosis is a device known as the "***X-Stop***." This device fits between the bony prominences in the middle of the lower back (spinous processes) and spreads them apart. This helps to increase the room for the nerves as they exit the spine. The X-Stop is not an option for many patients with spinal stenosis or patients with multiple levels of stenosis in the lower back.

While spinal stenosis is not likely to lead to paralysis if left untreated, it can have a limiting effect on an individual's quality of life. It is a very common problem that can be diagnosed with a simple test such as an MRI scan. If symptoms develop, primary care doctors are well-versed in identifying the possibility of spinal stenosis, and an appropriate referral can be made for further treatment.

When in doubt, check it out!

In situations that cause concern, or with the presence of pain, be sure to check with your primary care physician or orthopedist.

Infections as We Age:
How to Recognize the Symptoms and Learn How to Prevent Them
Bharat Motwani, MD

Which infections are more common among older persons?
Respiratory infections (e.g., *influenza*, *bronchitis* and *pneumonia*) and *urinary tract infections* (e.g., *bladder infections*) are common among older adults. In addition, infections of blood, skin and soft tissue are common in nursing homes. *Herpes zoster* (*shingles*), skin infections due to *bed sores* and *infections of surgical wounds* are some of the common skin infections. Also common are outbreaks of certain diseases such as *diarrhea* and influenza (flu).

What are symptoms of infections?
It is important to recognize that older people do not necessarily have the same symptoms as younger people. Infections in older persons might initially result in only a general decline in function, with the person not eating well, or perhaps falling. While they usually feel weak or sick, they do not always have fever. They might be lethargic or confused. Their white count might be high or low.

Why are infections more common as we age?
Infections are more common as we age for several reasons:
- The immune system may weaken with age.
- The body may respond more slowly to infections.
- It may take longer for wounds to heal.
- Nutrition might be poor.
- Other medical problems, such as diabetes, might be involved.

As the body ages, it undergoes some changes. Therefore, decrease in immunity and slow healing of wounds are normal, expected changes with aging. However, age by itself is not a risk factor for acquiring infections.

How can one prevent infections?

Infectious diseases account for one-third of all deaths in people 65 years and older. However, many infectious diseases are preventable. Some of the things that are helpful in preventing infection are eating healthy food to avoid nutritional deficiencies, practicing cleanliness (especially hand washing), exercising regularly and keeping immunizations updated.

What is the relationship between fever and infections?

Fever can be caused by infections. However, it can also be due to cancer or connective tissue disorders. Therefore, it is important to find out cause of fever before treating with antibiotics.

Which vaccines are advised for older persons?

Older people are encouraged to receive *influenza* (commonly known as flu), *pneumococcal* (commonly known as pneumonia), *tetanus* and *travel-related vaccines*.

What is influenza and why should older people be vaccinated?

Influenza (flu) is a common respiratory infection and a common cause of death in elderly. Also, older adults are prone to severe complications from this common illness because of co-existing chronic disease and weakened immunity. The single best way to protect against the flu is to get vaccinated.

306

What are the symptoms of influenza?

Flu usually causes headache, fever, chills, muscle aches, malaise, cough and sore throat. Most people recover fully within one week, but older adults may develop a persistent weakness that can last for many weeks and also face higher risk for developing complications, such as pneumonia.

Is the flu contagious?

Yes, it is highly contagious. It spreads easily from person to person, mainly when an infected person coughs or sneezes.

What types of flu vaccines are available?

There are two types of vaccines: *flu shots* and *nasal spray*. Nasal spray is not approved for adults 50 years of age or older. Therefore, in this chapter we will discuss only the flu shot.

How does the flu shot work?

The flu shot is an *inactivated vaccine* (i.e., it contains killed virus) which contains three influenza viruses. The vaccine is a shot, usually administered in the arm, given every year before the flu season begins. Because the flu season can begin as early as October and last as late as May, it usually is best to get vaccinated in October or November, but the shot can be given throughout the flu season. It takes about two weeks after vaccination for antibodies to develop in the body and provide protection against influenza virus infection. In most situations, one flu shot per year is sufficient.

How effective is flu vaccination?

The flu shot is 30-70% effective in preventing hospitalization and about 80% effective in preventing death from the flu.

Who should NOT get a flu shot?

People with an allergy to eggs, severe reaction to an influenza vaccine in the past or history of Guillain-Barré syndrome (a neurological condition) should not receive flu vaccine.

Why are seniors urged to get a flu shot every year?

Because the influenza virus changes every year, viruses in the vaccine are changed each year based on international monitoring and scientists' predictions about which types and strains of viruses are likely to circulate in a given year.

What are the possible risks from getting a flu shot?

Most people who receive a flu shot have few or no complications. Since the viruses in the flu shot are killed viruses, it is not possible to get the flu from a flu shot. The risk of a flu shot causing serious harm, or death, is extremely small. However, a vaccine, like any medicine, may rarely cause serious problems, such as severe allergic reactions. Possible side-effects include soreness, redness, or swelling where the shot was given, low-grade fever and muscle aches. If these problems occur, they begin soon after the shot and usually last one to two days.

Are flu shots covered by Medicare?

Yes, the cost of the flu shot is covered by Medicare. Many private health insurance plans also pay for the flu shot.

Where can I get a flu shot?

You can get a flu shot at your doctor's office or from other health care providers. You also may be able to get a flu shot from your local health department.

Is there any treatment for flu?

Yes, there is. But an anti-flu medicine has to be taken within 48 hours of onset of illness. Generally, if you get the flu, rest in bed, drink plenty of fluids and take medication such as aspirin or acetaminophen to relieve fever and discomfort.

What is pneumococcal disease?

Pneumococcal disease is a serious disease that can lead to *pneumonia* (infection of the lungs), *bacteremia* (blood infection), and *meningitis* (infection of the covering of the brain) and even death. The usual symptoms of pneumonia are cough with phlegm, shortness of breath and fever.

Why should seniors be vaccinated against pneumococcal disease?

While antibiotics such as penicillin were once effective in treating these infections, the disease has become more resistant to antibiotics. Therefore, prevention of the disease through vaccination is a smart thing to do.

Pneumococcal (NEW-moe-cock-uhl) vaccine protects against 23 types of pneumococcal bacteria which are responsible for about 80-90% of pneumococcal disease in the United States. Most people who get the vaccine develop protection within 2 to 3 weeks of getting the vaccine. While this vaccine prevents severe disease, hospitalization, and death in most people, it is not guaranteed to prevent all symptoms in all people. In general, pneumococcal vaccine is 50-60% effective in preventing pneumococcal disease and death from it.

Who should get pneumococcal vaccine?

All adults 65 years of age or older should get this vaccine. Shots are available at any time of the year.

Who should NOT get pneumococcal vaccine?

People who are pregnant should not get pneumococcal vaccine.

How is pneumococcal vaccine given?

It is administered ***intramuscularly*** (within the muscle) or ***subcutaneously*** (under the skin) as one dose. It also can be combined with other vaccines (by separate injection in the other arm) such as flu vaccine, diphtheria, tetanus, pertussis, and others.

How many doses of pneumococcal vaccine are needed?

Usually only one dose is needed. However, a second dose is recommended for those people aged 65 and older who got their first dose when they were under 65 if 5 or more years have passed since that dose.

Does pneumococcal vaccine work right away?

No. It takes about two to three weeks after vaccination for antibodies to develop in the body and provide protection against pneumococcal disease.

What are the risks of pneumococcal vaccine?

It is a very safe vaccine. Most side effects are mild, such as redness or pain where the shot is given. Less than 1% develop a fever, muscle aches, or more severe local reactions. Severe allergic reactions have been reported very rarely. As with any medicine, there is a very small risk that serious problems, even death, could occur after getting a vaccine.

What should one know about shingles?

Shingles is a disease that affects nerves and causes pain and blisters in adults. It is caused by the ***varicella*** virus, the

310

same virus that causes ***chicken pox***. The virus enters in the body as chicken pox virus and lies dormant inside nerves. As immunity decreases with age, the virus can reactivate to cause shingles. When started within 72 hours, treatment with anti-viral medicines can reduce the duration of rash and sometimes decrease the pain. Other treatment includes rest, avoiding stress as much as possible and eating well-balanced meals.

What are complications of shingles?

Pain (***post-herpetic neuralgia***) is the most common complication and can be debilitating. In some cases, ***blisters*** can become infected and ***scarring*** of the skin may result. If blisters occur near or in the eye, lasting ***eye damage*** or ***blindness*** may result. Some people may have ***hearing loss*** or a ***brief paralysis of the face***. In a small number of cases, ***swelling of the brain*** (***encephalitis***) can occur.

What is post-herpetic neuralgia?

After the rash of shingles is gone, some people may be left with long-lasting pain called ***post-herpetic neuralgia***. The pain is felt in the same area where the rash had been and can last for long time. The pain can be sharp, throbbing, or stabbing. The older you are when you get shingles, the greater your chance of developing post-herpetic neuralgia.

How is post-herpetic neuralgia treated?

It can be treated with ***pain-killers*** (***analgesics***), ***antidepressants*** (medicines to treat depression) and ***anticonvulsants*** (medicines to treat seizures)

Is shingles contagious?

Yes. While it is not possible to catch shingles from someone who has it, it is possible to catch chicken pox from someone with shingles.

311

What are symptoms and likelihood of contracting urinary tract infections?

Burning during urination, increase in frequency, urgency (feeling like one has to urinate immediately), pain in lower abdomen and fever are common symptoms of urinary tract infections. Women are more likely to get urinary tract infections than men because of their anatomy. Similarly, people with Foley catheters are more likely to get urinary tract infections.

What is asymptomatic bacteriuria?

As the name implies, *asymptomatic bacteriuria* means one has no symptoms of urinary tract infection but, when urine is examined under microscope, bacteria and white cell blood are found in urine. It is not uncommon to have asymptomatic bacteriuria in elderly patients.

How is asymptomatic bacteriuria treated?

Asymptomatic bacteriuria does not need to be treated. There is no advantage of treating it and there is no adverse effect if it is not treated.

Should seniors be concerned about HIV and other sexually transmitted diseases?

Despite myths and stereotypes, many seniors are sexually active. Drug use among seniors also is more common than people assume. Therefore, seniors are at risk of acquiring HIV and other sexually transmitted diseases just like anybody else. In United States, about 11-15% of HIV cases occur in people over the age of 50.

How can one prevent HIV and other sexually transmitted diseases?

Prevention is better than cure. Condoms, monogamous

relationships (limiting sexual relationship to only one partner who has tested free of all STD's) and ***abstinence*** help to prevent HIV and sexually transmitted diseases.

If you have questions about these or other conditions, please talk with your doctor or the local health department.

Eye Diseases of the Elderly
Ashok R. Penmatcha, MD

Diseases of the eye are among the most common ailments that affect adults. Many of us have heard of *cataracts, glaucoma, retinal detachments, macular degeneration,* and *diabetic retinopathy.* This chapter will discuss these topics to familiarize you with the diseases.

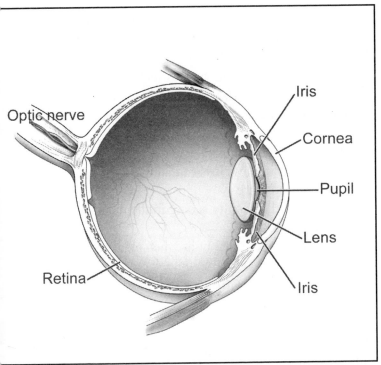

Figure 1. Normal eye anatomy (From NEI)

What is a cataract?

A *cataract,* described as a clouding of the lens inside the eye, is one of the leading causes of treatable vision loss in the United States. There are about 20 million Americans diagnosed with cataracts each year. This results in approximately 2 million cataract surgeries being performed annually. A vast majority of these surgeries result in significant improvement in visual function for the patient. Cataract surgery is one of the most successful interventions in medicine.

How do I know if I have a cataract?

A routine ***ophthalmologic exam*** includes an evaluation for cataracts. During this exam, the vision is checked under various lighting conditions. The lens in the eye is evaluated for any uncharacteristic discoloration and imperfections. The eye is also examined for any other disorders that may contribute to reduced visual function. Finally, your ophthalmologist will ask you how your vision is affecting or interfering with your daily life.

Some common symptoms include:
- Gradual painless loss of vision
- Increased glare
- Increased difficulty seeing in the distance
- Double vision
- Need for increased light when reading
- Poor contrast (for example, having difficulty tracking your golf ball across the blue sky)

What causes a cataract?

There are many factors involved and no one has a full understanding of the cause. However, there are some risk factors:
- Aging
- Family history of cataracts
- Certain medical problems like diabetes
- Certain medications like topical or oral steroids
- Trauma to the eye
- Ultraviolet light exposure

What are my options if I am diagnosed with a cataract?

Your ophthalmologist will discuss the options with you. Remember, a cataract is simply a clouding of the lens in the eye. If the clouding does not affect your vision, then in most cases the cataract will be left alone. It is difficult for your doctor to tell you how fast the cataract will change. Initially, a change in your glasses may be all that is needed to improve your vision to an acceptable level, or better lighting when reading or wearing sunglasses when driving.

If your ophthalmologist diagnoses a significant cataract and your vision has been bothering you, then it is a good time to consider cataract surgery. A complete ophthalmologic exam will be performed to ensure there are no other diseases that may be contributing to the poor vision. A general physical exam will also be recommended to assess your ability to tolerate outpatient surgery. If you are on blood thinners, your ophthalmologist will get permission from your primary care doctor to discontinue them for a few days prior to surgery. Since the cataract is actually in the lens of your eye, your lens will be removed and replaced with a small synthetic lens. Measurements will be taken in the ophthalmologist's office to determine which synthetic lens and power will be used to replace your lens.

Cataract surgery is typically performed as an outpatient procedure. The initial surgery is performed using a small pen-like instrument, which creates ***ultrasonic energy***. This energy breaks up the cataract into small particles, which are then removed by the same instrument. The new synthetic lens is then positioned inside the eye in the space previously occupied by the cataractous lens.

Do cataracts return?

Once the cataract is removed, the cataract does not return. However, the bag that the cataract was in is intentionally left behind after surgery to support the new lens implant. Over time, the bag may become cloudy enough to cause reduced vision or significant problems with glare. Your ophthalmologist will then recommend a laser surgery, called a *laser capsulotomy*. This is a quick painless procedure, usually done in the doctor's office, and visual recovery is rapid.

What's new in cataract surgery?

Historically, the new lens placed in the eye can focus only at one point. Most of the time, your surgeon will choose to correct your distance vision. Recently, *multi-focal lenses* have been developed to decrease the need for reading glasses. Some recent studies have shown that 80% of patients who had the new multi-focal lenses no longer required glasses for distance or close vision. However, this lens is not for everyone. Patients who may need excellent night vision and are concerned about glare do better with the standard intraocular lens. Also, patients with *astigmatism* may not be candidates for this lens.

Medicare and third-party insurance companies pay for most cataract surgeries as long as deductibles have been met. However, at this writing, the insurance companies will not pay for the multi-focal lens implant. This may contribute to a greater out-of-pocket expense for the patient.

What is glaucoma?

Glaucoma refers to progressive disease of the *optic nerve,* the cable that connects the eye to the brain. This disease has many different sub-categories; however, they share certain common features. These include *intraocular pressures too high for the continued health of the eye*, *atrophy of the optic nerve* and *loss of visual field*.

How does glaucoma affect society?

Glaucoma is a major cause of blindness in the United States. Approximately 5-10 million have increased intraocular pressure that is a risk factor for glaucoma. About 2 million have glaucoma, but only 50% know they have this disease. The cost of treatment and lost productivity amount to billions of dollars annually.

What are the two types of glaucoma?

There are two main classifications of glaucoma: 1) *open angle glaucoma* 2) *closed angle (narrow angle) glaucoma.*

What is open angle glaucoma?

Open angle glaucoma is a chronic, slowly progressive painless deterioration of the optic nerve. It shows a characteristic change in the optic nerve called "cupping" and visual field loss. Intraocular pressures are a risk factor. In general, the higher and more variable the pressure readings, the greater the risk.

How common is open angle glaucoma?

It is the most common form of glaucoma, making up roughly 65% of all glaucomas in the United States. Although it can be found in younger patients, it becomes particularly prevalent in ages greater than 50. The prevalence then increases with each decade of life. It is thought that at age 80, roughly 15% of the population may be afflicted with this disease. Glaucoma is more prevalent in the African American population, and the disease is more resistant to treatment among this population. Therefore, it is the number one cause of blindness in African-Americans.

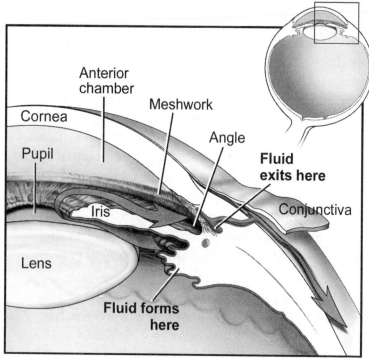

Figure 2. Poor outflow of fluid at the open meshwork can result in increased intraocular pressure (From NEI)

How do I know if I am at risk for open angle glaucoma?

Since open angle glaucoma causes painless and permanent loss of vision, it is difficult for a patient to know he/or she has this disease. Additionally, since central vision is often preserved until late in the disease, having 20/20 vision does not rule out the possibility of having glaucoma. This is why **full ophthalmologic exams should be performed every 1-3 years.**

What tests will an ophthalmologist perform in a routine glaucoma evaluation?

The evaluation will include a *review of family history*, a *full eye exam* including checking your vision, *examining the*

anterior and posterior segments of the eye. Special attention will be made to ***check the intraocular pressure*** as well as the ***appearance of the optic nerve***. Intraocular pressure in the eye is created by the continuous production of fluid in the eye. If this fluid is not allowed to drain effectively from the eye, the pressure builds. The higher the pressure, the greater the risk factor for developing glaucoma. Unfortunately, some glaucoma patients have normal pressures and some patients without glaucoma have high pressures. This makes the evaluation of the optic nerve the single-most important factor in diagnosing and following glaucoma. There are characteristic changes of the optic nerve that will point your ophthalmologist towards placing you into categories: normal, suspicious for glaucoma, glaucoma. Depending on the

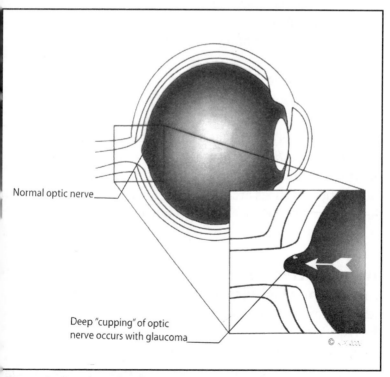

Figure 3. Cupping of optic nerve as a result of glaucoma

individual assessment, further tests may be ordered, including color photos of the optic nerve and visual fields.

What treatments exist for open angle glaucoma?

Treatment for glaucoma can range from *topical eye drops, oral pills, laser surgery*, and *trabeculectomy surgery*. All of these treatments benefit an individual by reducing both the total eye pressure from baseline and the fluctuation of eye pressure over time. No matter what the pressure was during diagnosis, it has been shown that a significant reduction in pressure can either halt or slow this disease. Medications either allow better outward flow of fluid from inside the eye or reduce the amount of fluid the eye makes. The choice of which medicine works best for an individual patient is made taking into account many factors:

- Side effects
- Effectiveness of the treatment
- Cost
- Ease of use

Laser surgery works by allowing better flow out of the eye. The laser is directed at the drainage system in the eye (*trabecular meshwork*) and through a complex reaction improves outflow. This procedure is simple and works for most patients. Risks are minimal. However, some patients do not get a good response and in others, the effect wears off in several years.

Trabeculectomy surgery

This surgery is limited to patients whose disease progresses despite more conservative therapy. Your surgeon will discuss the risks and benefits of this intricate surgery. The surgery involves creating a second outflow channel for fluid to leave the eye. The difficulty of this surgery arises from the fact that the body will try to close this surgical channel or the channel

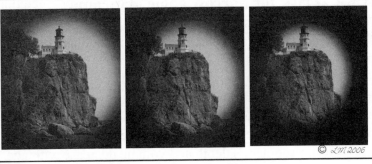

Figure 4. Vision changes over time with glaucoma

will work better than expected. Immediately after surgery the eye pressure can be too high, too low, or just right. Your surgeon will take steps after the surgery to help modulate the healing to make the surgery as successful as possible.

What is narrow angle glaucoma?

Unlike open angle glaucoma, narrow angle glaucoma typically presents with *pain, headache, pressure sensation, red eye, blurred vision* and *halos around lights*. This occurs because the eye pressures rise dramatically very quickly, from 15mmHg to as high as 70mmHg. The elevated pressure could cause permanent damage to the eye in a few hours to a few days.

Why does the pressure suddenly rise in narrow angle glaucoma?

Fluid is produced in the posterior segment of the eye but is drained in the anterior segment in the eye. In some people, the fluid causes the pressure in the posterior segment to increase relative to the anterior segment. This causes the iris to be pushed forward and drape over the drainage point in the eye, the trabecular meshwork.

Am I at risk for narrow angle glaucoma?

Your ophthalmologist will evaluate your eyes on each visit for this condition. Particular attention will be made for patients in the higher-risk category. It is most commonly seen in *farsighted* (*hyperopic*) individuals because they have shorter eyes. The shorter eye contributes to a more crowded anterior segment. Farsighted white women over the age of 50 are most at risk, especially if diagnosed with cataracts. The anterior segment's depth and volume decrease with age. Additionally, as the lens becomes more cataractous, the lens becomes larger, contributing to a more crowded anterior segment.

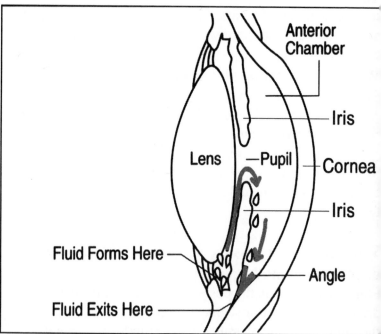

Figure 5. Narrow angle glaucoma (From NEI)

articular attention will be paid to the following during your xam:

- History of intermittent eye pain, redness, and blurred vision
- Medications
- Intraocular pressure
- Glasses prescription to look for hyperopia
- Cataracts
- Gonioscopy (a test which involves using a prismatic lens to look into the anterior segment to determine the extent of the narrow angle)

What happens if I am diagnosed with narrow angle glaucoma?

Based on a complete ophthalmologic exam, your doctor may explain that your drainage system is narrow but has not reached a critical level requiring treatment. In this situation, you will be warned of the symptoms to look for and will be urged to return immediately if they should arise. You will also be warned of some medications to avoid that can cause further narrowing.

The list below contains common and safe medications that in some cases of narrow angle glaucoma may cause further narrowing. These medicines DO NOT increase a person's risk for the most common type of glaucoma, open angle.

- Cold and sinus medications containing decongestants like pseudoephedrine (Sudafed)
- Medications for Parkinson's disease
- Antidepressants
- Medications for urinary incontinence (Detrol)

Is there a cure for narrow angle glaucoma?

Unlike open angle glaucoma, narrow angle glaucoma can be cured. If your ophthalmologist determines there is a critical narrowing or closure of your drainage system, a laser procedure can be performed. This procedure, called a **peripheral iridectomy,** involves creating a small hole in the iris far from the pupil. This hole helps balance the pressure in the anterior and posterior segments of the eye, preventing the forward movement of the iris and closure of the drainage system. This is an outpatient procedure that can be completed in minutes in most cases. However, those in complete closure can be more challenging. This is why your ophthalmologist may recommend this procedure as a precaution against complete closure.

What is a retinal detachment?

The retina is like the "film" in a camera. It picks up the light that enters the eye and converts it to electro-chemical energy and passes the information through the optic nerve to the brain. This layer gets blood supply from the retinal vessels and the back wall of the eye (**choroid**). The retina separates from the back wall of the eye and the parts of the retina that previously received blood from the choroid no longer get enough oxygen and die.

Most **retinal detachments** occur following separation of the vitreous gel inside the eye from the retina. The vitreous is a jelly-like substance that liquefies over time. As the vitreous degenerates, the liquid portion can quickly separate the remaining gel from the retina. This rapid separation can pull the retina and leave small holes. The liquefied vitreous can seep through the hole and get under the retina and pull it off (retinal detachment).

What symptoms will I have?

Early, when the vitreous first liquefies, all of us, as we get older, may see more **floaters**. When there is an acute vitreous detachment, patients may see a sudden increase in floaters. This results from debris from the separation floating inside the center of the eye. Flashes of light can also be seen during this period. The retina does not have any pain sensation.

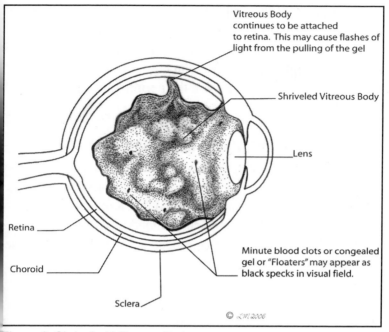

Vitreous Body continues to be attached to retina. This may cause flashes of light from the pulling of the gel

Shriveled Vitreous Body

Lens

Retina

Choroid

Sclera

Minute blood clots or congealed gel or "Floaters" may appear as black specks in visual field.

© *LM 2006*

Figure 6. Shriveled Vitreous Body

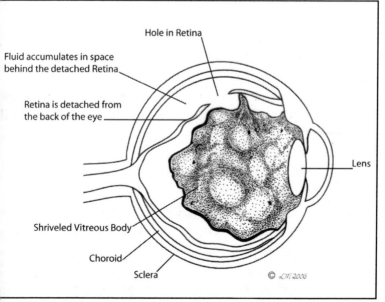

Hole in Retina

Fluid accumulates in space behind the detached Retina

Retina is detached from the back of the eye

Lens

Shriveled Vitreous Body

Choroid

Sclera

© *LM 2006*

Figure 7. Retinal detachment

However, if anything pulls on it like a separating vitreous, a flash of light results. The flashes may be initiated by movement of the eye because this causes the gel in the eye to move. A complete retinal detachment will cause a patient to see a dark curtain coming from the peripheral visual field to the center vision.

What treatment options are available?

Your ophthalmologist has many options to treat risk factors for retinal detachments as well as retinal detachments. If, following symptoms, it is discovered that a patient has high-risk holes, these holes can be surrounded with laser "weld spots." This is a simple office procedure, which can decrease but not eliminate the risk for retinal detachments.

If a retinal detachment is discovered, a retina specialist (ophthalmologist who did additional training) will use various techniques to remove fluid from under the retina and seal the hole. This surgery usually involves admission to a hospital and the repair is performed in the operating room.

Will my vision return to normal?

Retinal detachments, if not treated, can almost always lead to severe vision loss. Successful treatment may return vision back to normal in many cases, but many still have some level of vision loss. This is why it is important that treatment is begun as soon as possible, especially before the dark curtain approaches the central vision. Some patients need new glasses after the surgery because they may become more near-sighted. Others may need cataract surgery since the lens in the eye may become cloudier following a routine retinal detachment surgery.

What is age-related macular degeneration?

Age-related macular degeneration is the leading cause of

blindness in patients over the age of 50 in the United States. The *macula* is a small area in the retina that specializes in seeing colors and detail. Normal aging causes changes in this important area. Photoreceptors are reduced in density, cells lose natural pigment, and waste products accumulate under the macula. These aging changes only become problematic when they adversely affect visual function.

How do I know I have age-related macular degeneration?

Typically, patients do not know there is degeneration unless they experience vision problems. This can range from mild reduction in vision, poor adaptation to changes in lighting (long time to adjust from coming from a bright area to a darker-lit setting), wavy vision, and finally major loss of vision with central blind spot. A full dilated ophthalmologic exam will look for this condition. Your physician will evaluate your risk factors for this disease, including:

- Increasing age
- Hyperopia (farsightedness)
- Light iris color (blue eyes more at risk than brown eyes)
- Positive family history
- Cigarette smoking

If age-related macular degeneration is discovered, your ophthalmologist will place you in one of two categories: *dry macular degeneration* or *wet macular degeneration*.

Dry macular degeneration is characterized by slow loss of photoreceptors and the cells that support them. Instead of a normal macular appearance, this condition litters the macula with yellow spots and black scars. Visual loss is less severe and deterioration is typically slow.

Wet macular degeneration results from blood vessels from the wall of the eye (choroid) breaking through barriers to reach the macula. These blood vessels from the choroids are leaky and fragile compared to the retinal blood vessels. Eventually they will leak fluid and blood into the macula, resulting in severe distortion and loss of central vision. Your ophthalmologist routinely screens patients for this condition by checking the vision, checking for new distortions in the central vision with an *Amsler grid*, looking for new, unwanted blood vessels, fluid and blood.

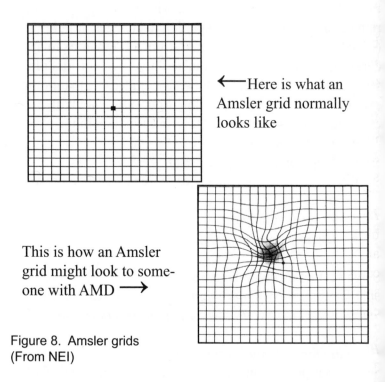

←—Here is what an Amsler grid normally looks like

This is how an Amsler grid might look to someone with AMD —→

Figure 8. Amsler grids
(From NEI)

What treatments are available if I am diagnosed with age-related macular degeneration?
Currently there are no treatments available for dry macular

degeneration. It is thought that light-induced and oxidative damage plays a role in accelerating the degeneration. Wearing sunglasses to reduce ultra-violet energy is likely helpful. Additionally, the chemical reaction of oxidation is thought to be important in aging; therefore, increasing antioxidants by using vitamins and quitting smoking may be helpful.

In a major study called the Age-Related Eye Disease Study, or AREDS, the National Eye Institute discovered that patients with intermediate or advanced macular degeneration can be helped with a specific high dose formulation of vitamins. This formulation of vitamins can be found in many national brands of vitamin supplements, all bearing the AREDS mark. This treatment cannot be expected to reverse macular degeneration but instead to slow its progression.

Wet macular degeneration has several treatment options, including *laser surgery*, *photodynamic therapy* and *injections*. These treatments are not a cure but can stabilize severe vision loss in some patients.

Laser surgery involves directing thermal energy to the bleeding and leaking blood vessel. If these irregular vessels are outside the center of the macula they may be treated causing regression. Unfortunately, the laser can leave a blind spot in the vision and sometimes the irregular blood vessels can return.

Photodynamic therapy uses a novel drug called *Verteporfin*. This medication is injected through an IV and circulates through the bloodstream. It also finds its way into the irregular vessels from macular degeneration. A laser light of specific wavelength is then directed toward the macula, activating the medication, causing the vessels to shrink. This procedure has the benefit of only damaging the irregular blood vessels and not harming normal tissue. This procedure also has limits since not all patients respond to the treatment as expected.

Injections of anti-blood vessel growth factors are the latest approach to wet macular degeneration. These new chemicals can cause regression of the harmful new blood vessels. Recent studies have shown some very positive results. Like the previous treatment modalities, there are downsides to this one as well. Not everyone will respond, the injections are very expensive, and finally it requires multiple injections into the center of the eye.

With advancement in technology and pharmaceuticals, macular degeneration in the future may become a manageable chronic disease like diabetes. Multiple treatment modalities may be used to help preserve vision for a lifetime.

What is diabetic retinopathy?

Diabetes causes slow and progressive damage to the blood vessels that nourish the eye. One of the most important and easily damaged parts of the eye is the retina. Its function is to convert the light that reaches the eye into an electrochemical reaction that is transmitted to the brain for interpretation. When the blood vessels are damaged, they leak fluid and blood into the retina resulting in less oxygenation of the tissue. Over weeks and months, these changes cause progressive loss of retinal function and vision loss.

Who is at risk for diabetic retinopathy?

All patients diagnosed with diabetes are at risk for this disease. Typically, the longer a patient has had this disease, the more likely retinopathy is present. This is why all patients need yearly screening eye exams. Once a person is diagnosed with diabetic retinopathy, the frequency of visits may increase if the disease worsens.

What symptoms will I have?

Initially, diabetic retinopathy may not be associated with any symptoms. Later, patients may experience slow vision loss. In later stages of the disease, patients may experience sudden onset of floaters and sudden loss of vision. Severe untreated disease can lead to a red, painful eye.

How is diabetic retinopathy detected?

A full ophthalmologic exam will look for complications related to diabetes. This includes the following tests:

- *Visual acuity*. Diabetes can cause reduced vision through a multitude of complications.
- *Refraction* (glasses measurement). Variations in blood sugars can change the power of your glasses.
- *Intraocular pressure*. Diabetic retinopathy can cause a type of glaucoma that increases eye pressure.
- *Examination of the lens*. Diabetics may develop cataracts at an earlier age.
- *Examination of the retina*.

How will the ophthalmologist examine the retina?

Using various lenses, your ophthalmologist will evaluate the back wall of the eye to look for characteristic changes. Your disease will be categorized into either *background diabetic retinopathy* or *proliferative diabetic retinopathy*.

Changes found in *background diabetic retinopathy* include:
- Weak-appearing blood vessels
- Fluid accumulation in the retina
- Retinal hemorrhage
- Retinal nerve damage

Changes found in *proliferative diabetic retinopathy* include:
- New fragile blood vessel formation in the retina
- New blood vessels forming on the iris resulting in a type of glaucoma

333

- Large vitreous hemorrhages causing floaters and severe vision loss
- Retinal scar tissue that can lead to retinal detachments

What treatment options are available for diabetic retinopathy?

Preventing complications from diabetes is the first line of treatment. Studies have shown that *improved control of your blood sugars* can limit damage associated with diabetes. Additionally, *well-controlled systemic hypertension and blood cholesterol* will also contribute to better prognosis. If you are diagnosed with diabetic retinopathy, your ophthalmologist will advise you on options available. If the retinopathy has not reached a critical level, a routine office follow-up will be advised. If critical diabetic retinopathy is diagnosed, then a thorough discussion of treatment options will be provided.

What is laser treatment in diabetic retinopathy?

Focal laser treatment for diabetic macular edema involves applying tiny laser burn spots to the areas around the macula. The macula is the most important part of the retina since it is responsible for most of our sharp vision. If it swells from leakage of blood vessels, the central vision may slowly and permanently deteriorate. Your ophthalmologist will take pictures of your retina with a special dye that highlights the blood vessels most responsible for the swelling. The laser is then directed at these weak blood vessels. The laser does not usually improve vision, but studies show that it reduces future vision loss by 50%. This procedure is done in the office and is painless.

Scatter Laser Treatment for proliferative diabetic retinopathy involves using the same laser, but the laser burns are much larger and greater in number. This procedure, unlike focal laser treatment, can be painful. Typically, after 1000-2000 laser spots, the irregular new blood vessels that have formed will shrink.

In some cases, laser treatment is not sufficient to stabilize diabetic retinopathy. Your surgeon may then recommend a *vitrectomy,* a procedure which allows the surgeon to remove blood and scar tissue from inside of the eye. Typically this is done in an operating room under general anesthesia.

Take good care of your eyes!

This summary of common eye diseases will give you a basic understanding of these conditions. Your ophthalmologist will give you and your family more detailed information during a consultation. It is important to have a list of questions available during your visit to sufficiently address your concerns and those of your loved ones. Further information can be found at various websites such as the *American Academy of Ophthalmology* (www.aao.org) and the *National Eye Institute* (www.nei.nih.gov)

We would like to credit the National Eye Institute, National Institutes of Health for the illustrations used in Figures 1, 2, 5 and 8 in this chapter.

Safe, Graceful Aging —
A Plastic Surgeon's Perspective
John M. Searles, Jr., MD
Anne R. Cramer, MD

People of all ages want to look their best. Here are questions that we frequently are asked by seniors.

As I have aged, I have noticed changes in my facial appearance. What are the usual signs of aging in the face and neck and what causes these changes?

As you age, you can expect *chronologic changes* in the face and neck. During the 30s, the *wrinkles* around the outer corner of the eyes appear and the upper eyelids can become redundant. In your 40s, you can look forward to the folds from the nose to the corner of your mouth becoming more pronounced and the vertical wrinkles above your nose and the horizontal forehead wrinkles becoming more noticeable. During your 50s, wrinkles appear in the neck and jowls along the jaw line begin to hang down, making the jaw line less distinct. After the fifth decade, the facial bony skeleton shrinks and the tissue deep to the skin atrophies, resulting in more wrinkles and sagging skin that is unevenly pigmented.

The above-mentioned changes are caused by factors that are independent of sun exposure and other extrinsic factors such as *smoking*, *alcohol abuse*, and weight gains or losses. As you age, skin will become less elastic, will lose underlying fat and bone stock and will develop abnormal pigmentation, which can be clearly made worse by the most important environmental factor: *sun exposure*.

What can I do short of surgery to slow down the aging process and to maintain a youthful facial appearance?

Over the last decade, there have been significant advances in a plastic surgeon's ability to improve upon the signs of facial aging without major surgery. One of the most popular, minimally-invasive procedures is injection of *soft-tissue fillers* to restore volume and fullness to skin in order to correct wrinkles and folds, such as the *nasolabial fold* (the line from nose to corner of the mouth) or the *glabellar creases* (vertical lines between eyebrows). *Restylane* is one such filler. It is safe, made of *hyaluronic acid,* which is a natural substance that already exists in our bodies. Studies have shown that it generally lasts for four to six months. A more long-lasting result is attainable with injection of one's own fat, but this is more invasive and often times has to be repeated multiple times to have a long-lasting effect.

A second popular minimally-invasive procedure is the injection of *Botox*. Botox injections are safe and can be used to improve the frown lines between the eyebrows, the "crow's feet" wrinkles near the outer corners of the eyes, forehead wrinkles which are horizontal and the folds that extend down from the corners of the mouth. Botox is a purified protein that temporarily paralyzes the facial muscles causing the above-mentioned wrinkles and folds. Placed correctly by someone familiar with the underlying facial muscles, it can not only rid one of wrinkles, but it can be used to shape (raise) one's brow position and to raise a down-turned corner of the mouth. Some of the best results occur when Botox is used in combination with Restylane.

Recently there have been major advances in the use of *visible pulsed light systems* and *nonablative lasers* to help with facial aging. The *Cutera laser* offers exchangeable heads that allow the skin to be targeted at different levels to treat *brown spots* and *photo discoloration* from sun damage, facial spider veins, wrinkles, and most recently, facial skin laxity. The treatments require no down time for the patient, do not require topical anesthesia, and are a real alternative to surgery in selected patients. The *Cutera Titan* utilizes safe infrared light to treat the dermis well below the outer skin surface. During the procedure, the skin's top surface is protected through continuous cooling that is built into the Titan hand piece. The most common areas treated are the jaw line, the neck and the abdomen. In selected patients, we have found it very useful to help tighten loosened skin.

What are the most important things that I can do to improve the health of my skin?

To prevent photo aging of the skin that leads to wrinkles, lines and a blotchy complexion, it is important to use a *sunscreen* of at least *SPF* (skin protection factor) 30 that blocks both *UVA* and *UVB* rays. Research has also shown that *antioxidants* (topical formulations of vitamins A, E and C) help combat the chemical reactions (*free radicals*) when skin is exposed to sunlight. When used with a good sunscreen, one has the best photo protection, decreasing the wrinkles and fine lines that characterize aging skin. Supplementing the body's natural supply of antioxidants with a topical treatment only makes sense and is supported by research.

Summary: Use antioxidants in combination with a sunscreen of at least an SPF of 30 that protects against both UVA and UVB light.

I love to tan, doing so year-round. During the winter, I use tanning beds. Do I have to worry about such behavior?

Yes, you do! The exposure of skin to UV light from tanning beds is cumulative and increases with age. Tanning makes you feel and look healthier, but it definitely will come back to haunt you down the road with more wrinkles and more discolored skin that sags much more than skin that is not photo damaged (that is, damaged by the sun).

More importantly, there is a direct correlation to sun exposure and the development of skin cancers. *Skin cancer* is the most common cancer in the United States, accounting for 1% of all cancer deaths. The three types of skin cancers are *basal cell carcinoma*, *squamous cell carcinoma* and *melanoma*. All of these cancers have an excellent prognosis if treated early, so it is very important to **seek medical opinion for any new or changing skin lesion**. Do yourself a favor and control the amount of sun exposure and use sunscreen with at least an SPF of 30.

Remember: Expose yourself to sun now, pay your plastic surgeon later.

I am 55 years old and had my eyes done 20 years ago. I am unhappy because I now look as though I have hollow, sunken spaces above and below my eyes. Is there anything that can be done for my appearance now?

It sounds as though you had an upper and lower *blepharoplasty* that removed too much of your eyelid fat. I bet you looked great for a while, only to look progressively more hollow and sunken as you aged. The trend today for eyelids is to minimize the fat removed in the upper eyelids, some surgeons only removing the excess skin. Often the amount of skin to be removed can be reduced if the brow is actually positioned higher through the upper eyelid incision (**browpexy**). With the lower lids, the fat is also handled conservatively to avoid a hollow look. Instead of being removed, the fat is transposed from deep to superficial and is sewn down over the upper cheekbone in order to give a full, youthful look. It may be possible to correct your hollowed look by injecting a soft-tissue filler, either your own fat or a Restylane-like product.

I have unwanted facial hair on my chin and upper lip, and also have spider veins on my legs that bother me. Short of electrolysis or painful injections of saline for the veins, is there anything that can be done for these problems?

The same laser that is used for facial rejuvenation can also be used for effective, long-lasting hair removal if the hair has pigment. The treatments are FDA-approved for all skin types and are permanent. Each hair goes through three stages: growth, regression and resting. The laser only works on hairs that are in the active growth phase. Since individual hairs will enter this phase at different times, multiple treatments are usually needed to give permanent reduction to hair follicles in a given area.

The *Cutera Cool-Glide* also can remove veins safely from different parts of the body on all skin types. Small facial veins and spider veins in the legs can be treated with great results in a safe, painless fashion. The laser delivers pulses of light energy, causing the vein to coagulate, and the blood is later reabsorbed by one's body. Often patients find one treatment sufficient, but sometimes further treatments are required due to the number and size of these vessels.

I am 55 years old, have had four children, and despite exercising religiously and watching my diet, I cannot get rid of my flaccid and redundant lower abdominal skin. Am I a candidate for a tummy tuck, and what is actually done during the operation?

If you are healthy of heart, do not smoke and do not have abdominal scarring from previous surgery that might compromise skin flap viability, you may well be a candidate for an *abdominoplasty*. During the operation, the surgeon makes a low, transverse incision just above the pubic bone and raises an abdominal skin flap off of the underlying muscles from pubis to lower breast bone. The belly button is preserved, circumferentially being excised from the skin flap. If the underlying muscle and fascia are loose, they can be tightened prior to excising the excess skin and fat. A new superior margin of the skin flap is sutured to the lower transverse incision and a new opening for the belly button is made and is sutured in place.

Liposuction would not be an appropriate option for you because it would most likely just make your skin sag more. It can, however, be used as an adjunct at the time of the abdominoplasty to help contour the abdomen and the flanks, but it needs to be done safely so that it does not interfere with the blood supply of the abdominal skin flap.

Remember: Tummy tucks are a no-no in smokers!

I am a 55-year-old-male and love to drink beer. I have a so-called "beer belly." Can this be treated by either a tummy tuck or liposuction?

Most males we have seen for either an abdominoplasty or liposuction of their beer bellies are not good candidates for ither. With the classic beer belly, the fat is actually intra-abdominal (that is, beneath the abdominal muscles) and cannot be removed safely. It can only be helped by dietary changes. If you don't want a six-pack abdomen, leave the beer in the grocery store.

Males do, however, tend to distribute their extra-abdominal fat in different areas than women, traditionally having a "spare tire" look, with fat accumulating circumferentially around their lower abdomen. This is a different picture than the classic beer belly, which is protuberant up high and tight as a drum due to all the intra-abdominal fat pushing outward on the abdominal muscles and skin. With the spare tire look, liposuction can be helpful if the man's skin has good tone and elastic recoil.

I am 55 years old and have always had large breasts, but for some reason they now are bothering me much more than previously. The bra strap grooves seem worse, upper-back pain is now almost always present and during the summer months I suffer from rashes and irritation beneath the breasts due to skin-to-skin contact. Am I too old for breast reduction surgery? How expensive is it?

First off, you are nowhere close to being too old. Some of our happiest patients are postmenopausal women who have similar problems from their large breasts. These problems can be resolved by breast reduction surgery, which usually also gives the woman breasts that she finds more esthetically pleasing and appropriate for her body size.

The surgery and related costs are most often covered by insurance companies. The process to determine coverage requires a letter, photos, and usually six weeks until determination by the insurance company is received. The operation is well-tolerated by most patients, usually only requiring an overnight stay. In our experience, the operation usually changes the woman's life for the better. Women who would not exercise become active, and most wonder why they waited to have their large breasts reduced.

Lately there have been important changes in terms of limiting the scars that are required to produce the reductions. These changes have been accompanied by higher levels of esthetic satisfaction in those patients who are deemed appropriate for such limited-scar surgery.

When treating women with large breasts, we have found that the major challenge is determining how small they want to be after the operation. It is frustrating for the patient to have to return for more surgery if her breasts are still too large and her functional complaints have not been improved. On the other hand, once it is gone, it cannot be replaced. Because of this, we always see our patients preoperatively multiple times to help the patient decide upon the size of her postoperative breasts.

With each pregnancy and as I age, I have noticed a loss of volume in the upper portions of my breasts. In addition, they have begun to sag. Do I need a breast lift, an augmentation or both?
If you are over 55, you have noticed these changes in your breasts for some time. Postpartum it is not uncommon for women to lose volume in their breasts and to have them begin to sag. The sagging can be made worse just by the intrinsic changes that our skin undergoes in terms of loss of elastic recoil as we age. What to do about such a situation depends upon how much sagging is present and where the nipple/

reolar complex is located. If the degree of sag is minor and
he nipple/areolar complex is above where the lower breast
omes off of the chest wall, a breast augmentation may be
nough to fill out the lax skin envelope and give the woman
hat she desires. The patient should understand that the
mplant will restore some of the upper breast volume but will
ot change the position of the nipple/areolar complex to a
reat degree.

'or those women who have more sag, some form of breast
ift will usually be required. Sometimes this can be done
vith the scars placed around the areolar complex. Other
imes they require scars (upside-down T) similar to those
equired for a breast reduction. The lift and augment can be
lone at the same setting, but it is usually wise to stage them.
The first stage is the breast lift to tighten the skin envelope
nd to raise the nipple/areolar complex. The second stage is
he augment to increase the volume.

am 60 years old and a survivor of breast cancer, aaving undergone a mastectomy over 15 years ago. Am I too old for breast reconstruction, and now is this done?

Good candidates for breast reconstruction are women who
ire healthy with realistic goals for restoring their breast and
body image. We have reconstructed breasts in women much
older than 60 years of age and found it to be a physically and
emotionally rewarding procedure.

The reconstruction can be done at the same time as the
breast cancer surgery or in a delayed fashion. Often times
surgery on the opposite breast such as a lift, reduction, or
augmentation will be done to improve symmetry of both
breasts. There are several techniques that can be used to
reconstruct the breast following a mastectomy:

1) Tissue expansion that stretches skin so that an implant can be placed at a second operation.
2) Flap techniques that use a woman's own tissue from either her abdomen (most common) or her back to create a new breast mound.

Flap techniques usually result in a more natural-feeling breast, whereas reconstruction with a tissue expander allows an easier recovery than flap surgery. The patient with a tissue expander will, however, have to repeatedly return to the office for three to four months to slowly fill the device to expand the skin. A second operation will then be needed to remove the expander and place an implant.

Regardless of the technique chosen, the nipple is usually created by small local flaps that can be done in the office under local anesthesia. This is followed by tattooing of the nipple/areolar area, also done in the office. Complete reconstructions usually require multiple procedures over several months time but dramatically improve a women's self image and quality of life.

If you are healthy, you are not too old!

Leaving the Hospital – How to Get the Care You Need
Jennifer Busch, LBSW

When will I leave the hospital?

When you are in the hospital, you are at an *acute* level of care. This means:

- The doctor needs to see you daily to make changes to your care.
- The care you are receiving can only be provided in a hospital.

Many factors determine when you will leave the hospital. The two major considerations are:

- When the doctor feels you are stable and do not need to be seen daily.
- When the medicines and care you need can be provided somewhere else.

What if I am too weak to go home?

If you no longer need to be in the hospital (*acute care*), then *skilled* or *transitional care* may be appropriate. *Skilled care* (also sometimes referred to as *transitional care*) is a means of obtaining additional nursing care and therapy so you can get stronger and go home. Many hospitals and nursing homes provide skilled care. Medicare does provide coverage for skilled care but requires a patient to meet certain guidelines to use these benefits. Most frequently, a need for *physical therapy* and an ability to work with physical therapy fulfill these requirements. Your need will be evaluated while you are hospitalized.

What if I need medical equipment at home?

If you need *medical equipment* and your doctor writes an

order, the ***medical social worker*** will obtain the equipment for you. There are many different providers of equipment in the area, and you may choose the provider.

Will Medicare pay for medical equipment?
Medicare Part B does pay 80% of the cost of *some* equipment as long as there is a doctor's order and the need for the equipment meets criteria established by Medicare. Many supplemental insurances will pay the remaining 20%. Medicare does not pay for dressing aids, reachers, shower stools and other items used in the bathroom.

What if I need help at home?
Services available to assist people in their homes include:
- A ***visiting nurse*** to assist with a medical need
- A ***home health aide*** to help with bathing
- ***Physical therapy***, ***occupational therapy*** and ***speech therapy***
- ***Homemaker service*** to help with household tasks
- ***Meal service***
- ***Shift care***
- ***Lifeline***

What will Medicare pay for?
Medicare will pay for a visiting nurse and a therapist if:
1. The doctor writes an order
2. There is a medical need
3. You are homebound

Medicare will pay for a home health aide if there is a need and the visiting nurse is coming. Medicare does not cover homemaker service, but the fee is often based on your income.

What is meal service?

Meal service delivers meals for people in their homes. There are several types of meal services. Some services deliver one meal at midday during the week and can provide frozen meals for the weekend. Other services provide several meals either weekly or every other week. Most diets can be accommodated. The costs vary depending on the service you choose. Your medical social worker can provide you the options and assist with arrangements.

What is shift care?

Shift care is a person or people who can come to stay with you for several hours at a time. There are several shift care providers in the area, and the cost varies. Medicare does not pay for shift care. If you feel you will need shift care, your medical social worker can provide you with a list of agencies and assist with arrangements.

What is a Lifeline?

Lifeline is a type of emergency-alert system that consists of a base unit attached to the phone line and a remote unit worn by the individual. The remote unit may be either a bracelet or a necklace and has a button to be used to summon help in an emergency. Many elderly people who live alone find this service beneficial. Medicare does not cover the cost of Lifeline.

Who can help me with these and other questions?

People leaving the hospital most commonly use some or all of the services described above. Should you have other concerns – finances, transportation, housing – it's important to know that the medical social worker at the hospital is available to assist and provide information. Please let a staff member know your concerns so the social worker can be contacted.

Financial Planning – It's Never Too Late to Start!
J. Clark Arons, FIC, CLU

> "*Left unto our own devices, when it comes to financial planning, we will do nothing.*" *Clark Arons*

Why should I worry about financial, retirement or estate planning?

Planning in one's life is very important. If we do not plan, the things that we want to accomplish usually do not happen. On the other hand, for some reason, *financial planning* is something that we just do not want to do! Financial planning reminds us of our mortality or our morbidity, and that is something that we do not want to face. It is easier for us to say to ourselves that we will do the financial planning tomorrow.

When we are younger, we do not worry about what will happen because we tend to consider ourselves immortal. After all, the accidents that we read about always happen to someone else; those accidents are never going to happen to us! The truth of the matter is, however, those accidents *do* happen to us, and if we want to control what happens to our estate and our families, it is important that we do the financial planning. The financial planning will assure our family that they will be taken care of in case of a debilitating injury or a premature death.

Retirement planning is an extension of our financial plan and is something that many of us wait until too late to do. If we want to know that we will be able to retire at a certain age and have our savings support us until our death, it is critical to have a retirement plan in place. Most of us do not worry a great deal about retirement until we are into our 40's, by that time, we may find that saving enough money for our retirement is difficult.

As we get older, our concern moves to *estate planning*. We wonder how we can ensure that our children will receive our accumulated assets without paying income taxes or estate taxes or probate fees. Estate planning helps us accomplish our goals of distribution of our estate to our heirs with as few fees and taxes as possible.

> *"I cannot advise that we remain as we are."* **Socrates**

What are the areas of a Financial Plan that I should be concerned about?

When we put together a total Financial Plan, there are three disciplines that we need to address: Legal, Tax and Financial To accomplish this, it is important to have a *legal advisor* (usually an attorney), a *CPA* or *tax advisor* and a *financial planner/advisor*. These three individuals will help you walk through the maze of questions and concerns that you have as you establish your plan.

Your legal advisor will help you determine which legal documents best fit your needs and your family's needs. The documents most often mentioned are *Will*, *General/ Financial Power of Attorney* and *Medical/Health Power of Attorney*. Depending on the value of your estate, your legal advisor may suggest that you consider a *Revocable Living Trust* (basically used to bypass probate), *Testamentary Trust* (usually used to establish a set-aside part of your estate for tax or legal reasons), *Irrevocable Life Insurance Trust* usually used to establish a sum of money that can be used to pay taxes or other estate transfer fees) or *Credit Shelter Trust* (usually used to aid in estate tax issues). There may be other legal documents that your legal advisor chooses to have you consider because of certain situations in your specific estate.

Of these documents, most people wonder why it is so important to have a Will. Your Will is usually the document that you put in place to establish the distribution of your assets at your death. The Will is also the place that you will name your:

- *Guardian:* the person(s) that you want to care for your children in case of your untimely death before the children are considered adults.
- *Executor:* the person that will handle the distribution of your assets at your death, or in case of a Will with a Trustee, the person that will close the estate and pass the assets to the Trustee.
- *Trustee:* if there is a Trust to be established, the Trustee will distribute your assets as the Trust directs.

Your *CPA* or *tax advisor* will aid in *tax planning*. The basic plan times are: working years, retirement, post-retirement and death. All of these areas may have specifics that your tax advisor wants you to consider. Your questions and statements will allow the advisor to assist you in the most appropriate areas. You may say, "I do not want to pay taxes at a higher income tax bracket when I retire than I do when I am working." Or you may ask, "How can I avoid paying taxes on my social security and pension when I retire?" These are both areas with which your tax advisor can help you.

"Worrying is like a rocking chair: it gives you something to do, but it doesn't get you anywhere." Van Wilder

Is one of the planning areas (Legal, Tax and Financial) more important than the other?

All of these planning areas are important and, put together in the correct way, a complete plan can protect your wants and needs for yourself and for your family. That being said, non of these areas of planning is more important than the other. The important part is the order in which they are done. Man legal, tax and financial advisors will tell you that the legal planning should be done first because that planning is the basis upon which the remainder of the plan is built. The lega plan will provide the Will, Trust (Revocable Living Trust or Testamentary, whichever your legal advisor recommends) and the Powers of Attorney (Durable and Health).

> *"All problems become smaller if you don't dodge them, but confront them. Touch a thistle timidly, and it pricks you; grasp in boldly, and its spines crumble."*
> **William Halsey**

How do I know that I will have enough money to live on through my retirement?

This is one of the questions that people ask the most! The problem is that sometimes they ask it too late. As you can imagine, individuals may have very different plans for their retirement, and the amount of money that they need at retirement may vary depending on what they want to accomplish. Someone who wants to live part of the year in a warm climate and the other part of the year in a cooler climate will need more money set aside than the person that simply wants to retire and live in one location. Certain individuals want to plan for a new car every four to five years, another family may want to plan an extended vacation or travel every year, someone else may want to work part time after they retire and yet another may want to do nothing but stay home and play with the grandchildren. Being able to support yourself and your family through retirement is a very important factor when you start to plan and set money aside for your retirement.

Many financial and tax advisors will recommend that you start setting assets aside for retirement as soon as you start working, no matter what age that is. A very important fact about retirement planning is not only how much that you set aside for retirement, but also the length of time that you have that money working for you. The compounding of the growth of your retirement savings will create substantial opportunities for growth in your retirement plan and the longer this money has to compound, the better off your financial retirement picture will become.

It is advisable for you to seek guidance from a qualified financial advisor to help you with your retirement plan. This advisor can help you decide which type of retirement plan best suits your situation and how to put that plan in place now and in the years to come. You will want to meet with your financial advisor at least annually to review the retirement plan and to see how the plan is progressing. By doing this, you will be able to stay on track with your retirement plan and make adjustments if necessary. Adjustments in the plan are likely to occur because your retirement needs may continue to change in the years to come. It is important that your financial advisor creates your plan with an inflation calculation so you will have the retirement funds needed based on the year that you retire, not the year that you started the retirement plan.

"Go to the edge of the cliff and jump off. Build your wings on the way down!" Ray Bradbury

What types of accounts are available for me to use for retirement savings?

As you can imagine, there are a plethora of accounts that may be used for retirement. There are some individuals who will qualify for certain accounts and not qualify for others. This discussion is not meant for taxation questions. The simple objective here is to talk about the types of retirement plans that are available.

It is a good idea for individuals to consider both pre-tax retirement savings and post-tax retirement savings. Pre-tax retirement savings are dollars that are deducted from your paycheck prior to you receiving your paycheck. These retirement savings will grow tax-deferred until you decide to take distributions from the accounts. *Some of the pre-tax plans that are available are as follows:

> Corporate Retirement Plans
> - 401K Plan
> - 403B Plan
> - 457 Deferred Compensation Plan
> - SIMPLE IRA Plan
> - Money Purchase Plan
> - Profit Sharing Plan
>
> Individual Retirement Plans
> - ROTH IRA
> - Traditional IRA
> - SARSEP
> - SEP
> - KEOUGH

Post-tax retirement vehicles are funded with dollars on which you have already paid taxes. Post-tax retirement opportunities are available in many different savings struments. Listed below you will find some of the options om which you might choose:

- Mutual Funds
- Annuities (Fixed or Variable)
- Stocks
- Bonds (Corporate, Municipal, Savings)
- Money Market Accounts
- Certificates of Deposit
- Savings Accounts
- Checking Accounts
- Commodities

ne of the keys to the growth of retirement accounts is e allocation of the retirement account. This means, very mply, the different type of investments that you have in e retirement account. You will want to visit with your nancial advisor as to the style of risk with which you e comfortable. Some people may be very happy with a onservative investment strategy, while others may want to e more aggressive in their investment strategy.

Note: The Internal Revenue Code (IRC) will be the guide s to what each individual can participate in as far as etirement plans are concerned, and the IRC is the document at explains the time limit that the pre-tax plans must be eld, without IRC penalty. The IRC will also explain at what ge individuals must start taking distributions from your pre- x plans.

"Well, all I know is what I read in the papers." Will Rogers

s it better to use pre-tax investments or post-tax nvestments in a retirement plan?

his is a question that will have varying answers depending

upon the individual who is asking the questions. The Internal Revenue Code (IRC) has certain restrictions that are placed on certain retirement plans because of income level, availability to a corporate qualified plan and other criteria. Your financial advisor and your tax advisor are the professionals that you will want to go to for an answer on th question. They are best equipped to help you walk through the tax laws and your individual situation as you compare th type of overall retirement plan that you want to design.

Another question that you will want to answer to help with this question is: At what age do you want to retire? This question will help you plan for retirement because it will he you understand which plan will accomplish retirement best for someone who wants to retire prior to age 59-½ or post a 59-½. If you plan to retire prior to age 59-½, you will want to make sure that you have access to retirement investments that have no IRC penalties prior to that age. This doesn't mean that you want to avoid pre-tax investments; it does mean that you may want to have both types of retirement investments, post-tax and pre-tax. If you do want to take distributions from your pre-tax retirement investments prior to 59-½ you can do so, but you will need to use a permissior that the IRC will give you, called equal *periodic distribution (72T)*. The explanation of this law is very detailed and you will want to consult with your tax advisor prior to making this type of choice.

Retirees may have a smaller income at retirement than they had during their working years. If this is the case, a pre-tax plan works well, because you can use the taxable retirement savings and not create a taxation concern because your income at retirement is not higher than your working income was.

358

> *"My chief want in life is someone who will make me do what I can."* Ralph Waldo Emerson

Why do I need to have Life Insurance after retirement?

Unfortunately, one of the biggest mistakes that we make when it comes time to retire is to convert our *life insurance* contracts to cash, or if the contracts are term life contracts we just let them expire or stop paying the premiums. Often there is a need to have the life insurance contracts in force long after our official retirement. What is important to remember is the reason that you had the insurance in the first place may have changed. The reason to have the insurance after retirement may be the same reason. There may be a word change in the offing at this time. Maybe you don't *need* the life insurance anymore; but instead maybe you *want* the life insurance. Of course this statement begs the question, "Why would I want life insurance at this time of my life?"

Let's take a look at a list of reasons that you may want to continue to own life insurance after retirement:

- Pay off debt
- Annuitize for extra retirement income
- Pay built-up income taxes in qualified plans (IRA's, 403B's, 401K's, SEP's, SIMPLE's, etc.)
- Pay estate taxes
- Establish a Legacy

There are other reasons that you may consider. Life insurance creates a supply of tax-free death benefit if it is properly set up. This will avail your estate the option to have tax-free cash available to use in case it is needed as your estate is distributed to your beneficiaries.

359

> **"Sometimes when you sacrifice something precious, you're not really losing it. You're just passing it on to somebody else."** *Mitch Albom*

Are there fees that I should be aware of that will be charged to my estate at my death?

The answer to this question depends on the value of your estate and the estate planning that you do in preparation for the distribution of your estate to your heirs. In a typical situation, there are five transfer fees that you need to be aware of and that you may need to prepare for:

- Probate
- Federal Income Taxes
- State Income Taxes
- Federal Estate Taxes
- State Inheritance Taxes

Most states will have *Probate codes* that must be met to close an estate. These codes will usually have fees associated with them, and the Probate fees will vary from state to state. The fees may be a percentage of the gross estate, or they may be a flat amount that is charged by an attorney to close the estate, or the executor of the estate may receive some payment for handling the estate. Some states will have maximum probate fees and some will not. Check with a local attorney to find the probate fees that will be charged to your estate.

Federal and state income taxes will be paid on the qualified plans that you own in your estate. These taxes will need to be paid prior to the distribution of the qualified plans to your heirs or your heirs will need to pay these income taxes. At this time, the federal income taxes could be as high as 35% and the state income taxes could run as high as the maximum tate income tax percentage. If the highest state income tax ate is 8.98% and the federal income tax rate is 35%, 43.98% f your qualified plans could have to be paid to the taxing uthorities prior to your heirs receiving any of that part of our estate. This may be one of the reasons that you *want* to ave life insurance after retirement.

ederal Estate Taxes are a work in process at this time and robably will be until the Congress acts on the current tax trata. This is a topic that would fill up several books if ve were to discuss it in detail. The way to prepare for this ituation is to plan for how your estate will be distributed at our death.

> *"The dictionary is the only place where success comes before work. Hard work is the price we must pay for success." Vince Lombardi*

low do I establish a Legacy for charity?

Many people will want to leave money to charity at their leath and some will want to set up an account that will keep n giving. This is often called *gifting in perpetuity*. This is imply setting an amount of assets aside in a Trust that will grow, and each year the income, growth or a percentage of he Trust account will be sent to charities of your choice. Basically the principal will stay in the Trust and the growth rom the Trust will be gifted. You can define the charities hat you want to receive these annual gifts or you can leave it up to the Trust to pick the charities.

These *Legacies* can be established in many different ways.
- Gift your qualified plans to a community foundation or a charitable trust at your death. A qualifying charity will be tax-free; therefore the income taxes

will not have to be paid.

- Establish a life insurance contract that will be placed in the community foundation or the charitable trust when it is written and either the community foundation or the charitable trust will be the beneficiary of the life insurance contract.
- Fund a community foundation or a charitable trust with part of your estate during your lifetime.

There are other ways to establish a Legacy, as you can imagine. Your legal counsel or your financial advisor will have options for you to consider.

The most important thing to remember is that if you have not already made arrangements with which you are comfortable, there are professionals who can assist you in your planning.

Transportation and Mobility Challenges Faced by Older Drivers

Denise A. Coiner, MS, RTR

Take a stroll . . . or maybe a *drive* . . . down Memory Lane!

Do you remember turning sixteen? Maybe, maybe not, but I would be willing to bet that **most of us remember** getting our very first driver's license! This ritual continues to represent those first steps to becoming an adult . . . an independent adult. Young people long for that square piece of plastic that gives them the freedom to connect at will to entertainment, food, companions, services . . . **freedom!** For so long they sit in anticipation for the day they can freely leave the nest with no strings, no questions, no worries. For years to come these same young people take flight day after day, year after year . . . and with the passage of time, these people, no longer so young, take the daily flight for granted, no longer getting the same thrill, but still enjoying the benefits of true freedom. But what happens when one day these once "young people" begin to notice that they aren't quite seeing the way they used to see?

Why do many older people hesitate to relinquish their driving privileges?

Ours is such a mobile society, and many seniors feel that driving helps them remain mobile and connected to their community, family and friends. Our private vehicles connect us to goods, services and activities which maintain our high level of independence. Just as it is exciting when we gain our independence by passing our first driver's exam, it can be unsettling when some older adults begin to experience driving challenges and fear losing independence.

What types of challenges are faced by older drivers?

Vision challenges

Aging eyes need more light to see, especially at night. The glare from oncoming headlights and wet roads also makes it very difficult to see. Aging drivers may realize that someone made the lettering on the street signs way too small! There are several diseases of the eye, such as macular degeneration and glaucoma, which can be triggered after the age of 60. Cataracts — which limit our visual field, reduce visual acuity and narrow our depth perception — are another common problem. This condition affects depth perception and results in the inability to discern the distance of oncoming traffic when making left-hand turns.

Hearing challenges

And as if this news wasn't bad enough, the hearing goes too! The cause could be as simple as years of build-up resulting in some major clogging, or the cause could be disease-related.

Reflex Challenges

Let us not forget the slowing down of the reflexes. As we grow older, we process information more slowly, affecting the way we react to changes in our environment on the road. This change in cognitive function directly affects our driving in heavily traveled areas such as major highways and, more specifically, during rush hour traffic.

Challenges with our muscles, joints and bones

As we age we are more susceptible to diseases affecting our joints, muscles, and bones. Osteoarthritis affects our flexibility and limits our range of motion in the neck and shoulder area. Diabetes can affect our muscles in the legs and feet, making it difficult to assess the amount of pressure we apply to the gas and brake pedal. Decreasing or erratic muscle strength might affect the maneuvering of the steering wheel.

Side effects from medications
The irony in all of this is that we as older adults recognize these changes and seek out professional help to soften the blow of many of these ailments. The doctors in turn prescribe medications to help us through these conditions and what happens? Side effects! Many drugs will affect our level of consciousness. Some may cause drowsiness or affect our reflexes, causing our driving abilities to be diminished. Let's face it: long periods of driving can become monotonous and can affect the alertness for anyone of any age. The addition of medication just makes it more challenging!

What steps can aging drivers take to maintain their ability to drive?
The picture may seem to look pretty grim at this point, but not to worry . . . there are a number of things that we all can do as aging drivers to prolong our years of mobile independence.

Limit unnecessary distractions
For starters, everybody, young and old, can limit the amount of unnecessary distractions. Turn down the radio and don't talk on your cell phone or program car gadgets while on the road. And if you can't engage in conversation with your passengers and keep alert to driving situations, then just don't get involved in conversations while driving.

Have vision and hearing checked regularly
It is important to have your vision checked often. Many diseases of the eyes are correctable. Having your vision checked often may result in something as simple as new corrective lenses or minor surgery. Hearing checks may also

result in a good cleaning of the ear canal or a simple aid to help you hear better.

Understand that our reaction time slows as we age

As we age, our reflexes are slower. We process informatic more slowly, which in turns affects our ability to react to driving situations. Limiting driving in heavily traveled are such as major highways and at busy times of the day (e.g., rush-hour traffic) is advisable.

Focus on physical and mental well-being

Keeping mentally alert and physically fit will help. Join a senior exercise group and challenge yourself to be more flexible, or take up a sport such as golf or swimming, which will strengthen muscles and flexibility. Know the medications you take and the side effects they may cause. The use of antihistamines, antihypertensives, or antidepressants increases driving risk because they can cau drowsiness; some can also cause hypotension or arrhythmi Some drugs, such as muscle relaxants and stimulants, may alter sensory perception. Check with your physician to ma sure the drugs you take will not adversely affect your drivi ability. If you are taking any of these types of medication arrange your schedule so that your driving doesn't coincid with the onset of the side effects.

Strategize to avoid challenges faced by many aging driver

Researchers have found that the most frequent accidents ar caused by failure to yield, making left-hand turns and runn stop signs. Being aware of these might make you more cautious when you drive. Also, if you feel stressed driving night or during busy times of the day, try to limit and avoic these circumstances.

Brush up on and update our driving skills

There are other options to keep us on the road as well. Wov

driver's education for the graying populations! We may think this is NOT for me: "I have been driving for fifty years; why do I need driver's education now?" The reality is that older drivers do have one big advantage over the younger drivers: Experience! However, learning how to drive with some of the aforementioned challenges might be just what is needed to keep your driver's license.

AARP, one of the largest organizations for older adults, has a well-respected driver education program that it offers in conjunction with local community colleges and senior-service programs . . . and taking it might also decrease your insurance premiums! In addition, several other organizations offer driver education programs to help with taking the driver's test again. Just check with your local Department of Motor Vehicles to learn about the programs that are offered for seniors.

Some states are looking seriously at changing their system of license renewals. Some states already have requirements in place to retest drivers over the ages of 70, 75, and 80. One recommendation is that a more uniform and stringent system of license renewals be adopted by state legislatures. These rules would not just address the unique problems posed by the elderly driver, but drivers of any age.

Automobile design also might change, with systems designed specifically to aid seniors. A downfall to this might be the new technology itself, since you would have to *learn* the new technology, requiring you to multitask to activate the new system.

Speaking of new technology, if you have Internet access, there are many Websites devoted to elderly drivers. Some have tests you can take online to assess your driving ability. There is also a wealth of information to keep you informed about changes in road rules, directions, etc., such as what to do in certain circumstances and sign recognition.

Statistics show that by 2020, there will be about 40 million drivers over the age of 65. We are not all going to age the same, just like we didn't all mature the same. We must still be responsible and know when it is time to quit driving or, at the very least, know when it is time to seek some assistance.

What types of transportation options are available for non-driving seniors?

If, after you have read this, you decide that maybe it is time to pass your car keys down to your grandson, you may be wondering what options are available to you. Well, if you live in a metropolitan area, your options are more numerous than if you live in the rural areas. However, either way, it is going to take a little detective work on your part to find out what your options are.

You can start by contacting your local Area Agency on Aging, health departments, community resources, churches, hospitals, senior centers and other senior-service organizations. They will be able to put you in touch with the appropriate transportation professionals to help you get where you need and want to go.

One last point: Don't forget your children!! If you are lucky enough to have them living nearby, remind them of all the times you drove them places before they got their driver's license. They should be more than happy to help you out!!

Research and the Mature Adult
Penny Stoakes RN, CCRC

"It is one of the most beautiful compensations of life, that no man can sincerely try to help another without helping himself. – Ralph Waldo Emerson

We frequently hear and see news about possible cures for diseases. Have you ever wondered how these new medicines, devices or cures are found? Would you be interested in participating in a project that could change the face of medicine? You could have a vital role in making medical history – if not for yourself, then for your children, grandchildren and generations to come. There are many rewards and challenges of participating in *clinical research*. This chapter explains some basic information of how to become involved in *medical research*, and how to ensure that you are participating in a safe, FDA-controlled clinical research trial.

Participating in a clinical trial requires a time commitment, as well as the knowledge that not all people will benefit from the treatment. The greatest reward, however, is the knowledge that you are participating and helping to provide new information that will contribute to the care of future patients of the same type of disease process you are experiencing.

The following question-and-answer format can help you decide if participating in clinical research is something you might like to do.

What is a clinical trial?

A ***clinical trial*** is a well-thought-out plan or blueprint (often referred to as a ***Protocol***) with defined goals and objectives. It most often utilizes a new drug or device believed to improve the existing treatment. Sometimes it is a treatment for something for which there is no known cure. In some instances, there may a possible new use for an already existing product. In all clinical trials involving experimental drugs or devices, this plan must be presented to the FDA (The Food and Drug Administration, an agency of the federal government.) This plan must have specific goals, including the type of patient and type of disease process that is being treated. There are also endpoints and safety mechanisms in place that protect the human subjects. There are many rules, and all are rigidly enforced; high standards are maintained. The study records are precisely maintained frequently, not less than quarterly. The doctors participating in the research sign a legal document attesting that they accept the responsibility for the conduct of the trial, and for other medical professionals who are assisting in the trial with them. Clinical trials are almost always sponsored by pharmaceutical or device companies, and sometimes by physicians who have ideas about improving existing treatments.

There are several phases to a clinical trial.

- Phase I usually tests the appropriate dose of medication and determines both how this drug distributes itself in the human body and how it is eliminated. A small number of subjects are enrolled in this Phase, typically healthy volunteers.
- Phase II usually tests the safety and, to a lesser extent, the effectiveness of a drug or a device in a larger number of patients.
- Phase III is a very large study that is performed prior to releasing the drug to the market; predominantly, it tests the effectiveness and safety of a drug or

device. Data from Phase III studies are submitted to the FDA to allow the release of new drugs or devices to the market.

Why would I want to participate in research?

Participating in research is something that you should feel comfortable doing. You should enjoy participating in a trial and never feel threatened, coerced, or at risk. You will have access to the latest technology in drugs and devices, something to which you might not have otherwise. You also are subject to receiving a *placebo*, which is a medication "look-alike" but without any active drug in it. Occasionally, clinical trials need to compare results against a placebo arm in order to measure effectiveness. Most of the time you will be "randomized," much like the flip of a coin, to the type of treatment you receive. The treatment you receive is "blinded," meaning you, your doctor or your study coordinator will not know what you're getting until the study is completed. In the unlikely event that you would have any problems or a complication, there is a way to unblind or identify the treatment you have received. If at any time your doctor thinks the treatment is harmful to you, you would be removed from the trial.

Who pays for the study treatments?

Clinical research sometimes involves additional tests and follow-up visits not covered by insurance. This usually is funded by the sponsor, foundations, hospitals or governmental agencies. Ask questions about who pays for these additional tests, and make sure you have who is taking care of the bills in writing. You should have a phone number of the clinical coordinator you can call and talk to in person to resolve any issues quickly. You should not have to pay any out-of-pocket expenses to participate. Most likely, you will get exceptional follow-up care when participating in a clinical trial.

How is my identity protected?

It is your right as a research subject to have all your personal health information and identification protected. Precautions are taken to maintain confidentiality and security of study records at all clinical sites. Paper-based records will be kept in a secure location and will be accessible only to personnel involved in the research project. Computer-based records will be password protected and will be accessible only to personnel involved in the research project. All members of the research team are required to sign statements agreeing to protect the security and confidentiality of the research participants. Whenever feasible, identifiers such as name, social security numbers and date of birth will be removed and replaced with a study number.

What is an Informed Consent?

Never participate in research without signing a consent form. An ***Informed Consent*** is the process of learning about the trial. It is based on three elements:

> 1) Complete information about the research study. This will include the name of the study doctor, how to reach him or her and who is sponsoring the research.
> 2) A complete explanation of why you are being asked to participate in the trial and what is expected of you when participating, as well as risks and benefits of the proposed treatment. This would include the length of time involved and how many visits and tests may be required.
> 3) Explanation of the participation being strictly voluntary in nature. You should never feel pressured to participate if you are not comfortable doing so.

You should only participate in clinical research if you are comfortable with your doctor and the research coordinator

nd you are willing to fulfill the time obligation. You may
lways withdraw your participation if you feel uncomfortable
r if your doctor feels there might be a safety risk, but the
esearch needs to be completed in order to validate the
utcomes.

esearch participation can be a richly rewarding experience,
specially with the knowledge that you might very well help
hange the history of medicine.

How to Talk to Your Doctor!
Suzy Hartung, BA

There's been kind of a "sea change" in our society's perception about how to communicate with our health care providers.

Whereas doctors used to be widely thought of as remote authority figures, there is an increasing emphasis in our society, by doctors and patients alike, on *patients being active partners in their own health care*.

This certainly doesn't mean that doctors should do anything less than usual; it actually means that patients need to do more than usual! Rather than having a system in which patients put themselves in "neutral gear" and wait passively for doctors to ask the right questions, make diagnoses and order prescriptions and other interventions to "make everything better," many doctors today believe that the most effective health care system involves patients being alert to their own bodies and communicating proactively, clearly and concisely with their doctors.

How can I "set the stage" for a successful appointment?

- **Plan ahead!** Prepare a list of concerns and health information *(see below, "What do other doctors suggest is the most effective way to communicate with our doctors?")*. Because we have a limited amount of time when talking with our doctors, we need to make each second count. Making a list is an excellent way to make sure we have all the info we need to "present our case" to our doctor.

- **Get reinforcements!** If possible, have a family member or friend go into the exam room with you so that you'll have an "extra set of ears." They, too, will hear what the doctor says, take notes, remind you of important information to share with the doctor, etc.

- **Know what you need, as well as what you can and cannot do!** If you are asked by the medical assistant, nurse or doctor to do something you have great difficulty doing or simply are unable to do (e.g., sitting on the exam table if you have trouble keeping your balance), by all means, **say something**! Your doctor and his or her staff won't know unless you tell them!

- **Think ahead, and be part of the solution.** If you know ahead of time that something will be difficult or impossible for you, try to figure out an alternative before arriving at your appointment. For example, "I'm sorry. I can't sit on the exam table to have my blood pressure taken, but if we can pull this chair close to the exam table, I could sit in the chair. Would that work for you?"

- **Sound off!** If you have a concern about something, be sure to let the doctor know. Or if you don't understand something your doctor has said, ask for clarification.

What do other doctors suggest is the most effective way to communicate with our doctors?

Much has been written in the past several years about the most effective means of communicating with our doctors. One of the most interesting, helpful and humorous books is **YOU: The Smart Patient**, by *Michael F. Roizen, M.D.*, and ***Mehmet C. Oz, M.D.***, in conjunction with ***The Joint Commission on Accreditation of Healthcare Organizations (JCAHO)***. Doctors Oz and Roizen are frequent guests on the ***Oprah Winfrey*** show; perhaps you've seen them there and have learned good tips about taking better care of ourselves. I strongly encourage the purchase of this book, as well as their first book, **YOU: The Owner's Manual**.

Doctors Roizen and Oz encourage patients to prepare two lists and keep these lists with them at all times:
- *notes listing current concerns*
- *a basic health information sheet*

These doctors urge patients to bring both of these lists to their doctor appointments.

List #1: What do doctors want to know from their patients – a/k/a, "What brings you here today?"

Doctors Roizen and Oz urge patients to be ready to answer the following questions about any situation that concerns you enough that you are bringing it to the doctor's attention:
- What caused this?
- When was it diagnosed?
- How are you treating it?
- Has it gotten better or worse?
- When did it first begin to noticeably improve or worsen?
- What makes it better?
- What makes it worse?

When the patient has thought through this information and jotted down a list, that helps the patient get on the same "wavelength" as the doctor, be more focused and provide more accurate, helpful information to the doctor. By the

patient following this practice prior to the appointment, both
the patient and the doctor will be able to make better use
of the time available during the appointment. And, since
patients sometimes become flustered or nervous when in a
doctor's office, having a list is a good "back-up" to ensure
that the really significant information will get shared with the
doctor.

List #2: What should the health information list include?

- **Name, address, phone number(s)**
- **Current health conditions** (either in order of the
  challenges they cause in your life or alphabetically;
  who, if anyone, is treating you for this if different
  from primary care physician; when diagnosed, if
  you know)
- **Other health history** (prior surgeries, diagnostic
  procedures & approximate date; if you know the
  results, list them following the procedure)
- **Allergies to medications** (on my list, I place this
  entire section in red to highlight it)
- **Current medications** (name of medication and
  dosage; be sure to include any over-the-counter pain
  medication, vitamins or minerals you take)
- **Personal information**
- **Date of birth**
- **Blood type** (if you know)
- **Primary care physician** (name, address, phone
  number)
- **Other doctors who are treating you** (name, address,
  phone number)
- **Insurance information** (name of insurer, insurance
  ID number, phone number that is listed on the
  back of your card)
- **Pharmacy** (name, address, phone number)

- **Person(s) to contact in case of emergency** (local, out-of-town contacts – name, their relationship to you, phone numbers, identified as daytime, evening or cell)

o we have any examples of "health information sts" being effective?

s a personal aside, I will share with you that I have llowed this practice of preparing comprehensive health-formation lists for approximately 10 years and have found to be very helpful. Because I have and manage several ealth situations that can be rather challenging (multiple lerosis, fibromyalgia, asthma, hypertension, etc.) and ecause I occasionally am unable to speak clearly if one r more of these conditions is "flaring," I make sure that I ave everything in writing that health care providers need to now to treat me. This has been very helpful both in urgent tuations, such as being a patient in an emergency room ithout any family or friends present, as well as in "routine" ealth care appointments – although many of us who are ot in the field of health care probably do not view ANY ppointment as "routine"!

began this practice while I was working and living in urope, during which time I had these forms translated into everal additional languages, and I continue the practice to his day. All of my providers find the sheets helpful, and ''s a good checks-and-balances system for me, as well, ecause I can refer back to my notes quickly if there ever is question about what I reported or when I reported it. And, s a "bonus," I feel organized and confident that I have done vhat I can do ahead of time, which allows me to be more omfortable in health care settings. Spending a little time reparing and copying the personalized information sheet s a small price to pay for having peace of mind, especially in times of stress or emergency. My family and friends also tell me that they are relieved that I always have this information sheet available; in fact, I also give them copies … just in case. And then, being prepared, I just go on with my "normal" life!

Now, as part of my community volunteer work, I help senio develop such forms, printing copies for them as well as giving them the document on a diskette. This makes it easie for them or friends or family to update the information shee when necessary.

What is the "File of Life" and how can it help m or my loved ones in times of emergency?

Many of our local communities encourage seniors to keep updated health information sheets in red vinyl "*File of Life*" magnetized pouches on our refrigerators. There also is a smaller, non-magnetized version that can be placed in one's billfold. Our local and regional first-responders (EMT's, firefighters, police) all are trained to look immediately for "File of Life" pouches on refrigerators or in billfolds. There also is a new system that the Sheriff's department and the local TRIADs are promoting, the "Yellow Dot" program, whereby people place a yellow dot on their rear window to indicate that there is emergency information in their car's glove compartment. I strongly encourage your participation in the "File of Life" and "Yellow Dot" programs. Contact Senior Voice, your Sheriff's department or your local Area Agency on Aging for more information.

What are other ways I can plan for emergencies?

No one likes to dwell on negative thoughts, but it's smart and positive to prepare for emergencies … just in case. Key documents that we all should have within easy reach include
- *Place healthcare information sheet / red "File*

380

of Life" pouch on refrigerators and in billfolds and glove compartments: In fact, you can just fold one of the information sheets discussed above and place it in the red magnetized pouch on your fridge and the small red pouch in your billfold. *(See above, "List #2: "What Should My Health Information List Include?")*

- *Insurance and Medicare cards*
- *Driver's license or other photo I.D.*
- *Emergency (disaster) plan* that you and your family have developed. Both the American Red Cross (www.redcross.gov) and the U.S. Department of Homeland Security (www.dhs.gov) provide helpful information on their Websites.
- *Advanced Care Planning:* It is essential that we think through our preferences regarding how we want to be treated through the end of our lives, discuss those preferences with our families, and record those preferences in writing so that they are available to medical care facilities and personnel, our families and our legal counsel. In the Iowa and Illinois Quad Cities, Generations Area Agency on Aging, Genesis Health Systems and Trinity Health System are working collaboratively on such a project, called "Choices Connection." For more information, contact any of the three partner agencies listed above; trained volunteers are available to help you fill out the paperwork once you have decided your preferences.

What are the benefits of becoming more of a partner in our own health care?

It's essential that we all become advocates for ourselves. The information discussed above will help us be more secure that all of our "regular" doctors, as well as emergency providers and family, have clear, accurate, updated information about us.

Again, we need to remember that WE are in charge of our health and well-being; doctors and first-responders will help us with their technical expertise, but for as long as we are able, it's important that we remain focused and "proactive" in making decisions that help us live healthful, positive and fulfilling lives at all stages of our lives.

If you need help to start developing your health-information list, feel free to contact the Retired & Senior Volunteer Progr (RSVP) of Eastern Iowa & Western Illinois (309.793.4425; shartung@wiaaa.org). We'd be happy to help you get starte ... and you'll feel ... and BE! ... so much better-prepared!

How to Engage in Positive, Graceful Living and Aging:
Remaining Engaged in Your Community Can Also Enhance Your Own Well-being!
Suzy Hartung, BA

fore getting into the "heart" of this chapter – how to
ain engaged in our communities and why volunteering is
helpful and healthful for us as we age – let's explore a few
ic concepts.

- Although we're all getting older, minute by minute, many of us do not think of ourselves as a "***senior***" or as "***elderly***." As a society and culture, we need to rethink our vocabulary and our approaches to aging.

- "***Aging***" is not a static state of being at which one arrives at an appointed time. Aging is, instead, an integral part of life – a continuum, an ongoing process of living our lives as fully as we can, from our earliest days to our final days.

- "***Graceful aging***," as reflected in the title of this book, flows naturally from "***graceful living***." We will take a look at what graceful living and graceful aging can mean in terms of enhancing our lives.

- There does not have to be a dramatic "line of demarcation" that we cross from non-aging to aging. ***Principles of healthful and harmonious living apply to people at all ages.*** Individuals and society as a whole benefit from people being ***conscious, focused and intentional in living lives of dignity, integrity, gratitude and joyfulness at all stages of life and at all ages***.

- Older adults often have a strong sense of what psychologist ***Erik Erikson*** labelled as ***Generativity***: a stage in adult development in which people unselfishly give "the gift of self" to family, friends, sometimes strangers and their community. Often there is a strong sense of nurturing and wanting to "give back" and nurture the development of community.

- Each day is a new opportunity to seek joy and love and bring it to others. As poet *Anne Morrow Lindberg* wrote, "The seeds of love must be eternall resown."

What does it mean to be a "senior"?

As a *"Baby Boomer"* who works with seniors my age (60) and older, I know how challenging it is to develop a profile a *"senior."* Older people no longer are easily pigeon-holed into one neat box . . . and, truth be told, they probably never were. They – *we!* – might be anywhere on the *continuum of aging*: being strong and active, then becoming less active eventually becoming more frail.

In my organization – the *Retired & Senior Volunteer Program*, or *RSVP*, sponsored by *Western Illinois Area Agency on Aging* – we recruit and place senior volunteers in community programs and agencies. We currently have more than 1000 volunteers assisting more than 130 not-for-profit or governmental organizations. Last year our volunteers provided more than 146,000 hours of service to their respective communities! Since the age of our volunteers ranges from 55 to 98, a 40-year age range, there's no way we can quickly describe or profile a "senior" when he or she could fit anywhere on that 40-year continuum. So . . . we have to update our vocabulary and our approach to "seniors."

How do we go about redefining mileposts in the aging process and updating our vocabulary?

In the RSVP program (which has been active nationally

ce 1969, through an amendment to the Older Americans
t of 1965, and locally since 1974), we are learning that
r more traditional approach to recruiting senior volunteers
not particularly interesting to or effective with Boomers.
erefore, we, along with millions of other people in our
tion, are embarking upon a new journey in understanding
e aging process and redefining mileposts in that process.
e are, indeed, *"making the path by walking."* As we
ep moving on this path, we are developing *new ways of
oking at aging*, *new vocabulary* (that is, new terms for the
ileposts that we discover) and *new ways of approaching
d engaging "seniors."*

hat does the term "graceful aging" signify?

e title of the book you are reading, with its focus on
iraceful Aging," is both interesting and provocative. While
me older persons resonate with the concept of *graceful
ing*, others sometimes resist the term "graceful," assuming
at this refers only to those who are blessed with physical
ace. However, that is not the intent of this term.

rst, "aging" is not a static state of being at which one
rives at an appointed time. *Aging is an integral part of
fe* – a continuum, an ongoing process, not a static state of
eing. It is important not to deny it but to embrace it and be
harmony with it!

herefore, *"graceful aging" flows naturally from "graceful
ving."* At all stages of our lives, we do well to consciously
xplore the following questions and refine our answers as our
rcumstances change:

- What makes our lives meaningful?
- How do we continue to weave threads of
  meaningfulness and integrity throughout our lives,
  adapting (hence the concept of *gracefulness*!) as our
  situations change?

385

- How can we maintain as high a quality of life as possible?

What characterizes "graceful living" and "graceful aging"?

- *Living in harmony* with ourselves, our circumstance our surroundings and those around us.
- *Determining what's appropriate to expect of ourselves* and tweaking or fine-tuning these expectations as our circumstances change.
- *Communicating* those expectations to others. We can train others to learn what is appropriate to expect of us. And it's much more enjoyable when expectations are communicated to and understood by others. *Dissatisfaction* occurs when there is a "disconnect" between what we expect and what we encounter, while *satisfaction* occurs when there is "harmony" between what we expect and what we encounter. Therefore, making expectations clear, both for ourselves and others, enhances the satisfaction and harmonious interaction of everyone involved.
- Finally, "graceful living" and "graceful aging" involve *taking responsibility for our own lives and situations* – health, finances, relationships, happiness and well-being – and "gracefully" and graciously adapting as our situations evolve.

How can we maximize our health and well-being as we age?

In addition to the excellent suggestions that have been made in the preceding chapters of this book, it is essential that as we proceed on our life journey, we are *conscious, focused and intentional about respecting life, finding and expressing joy, and living in wholeness and integrity*. For

386

ose of a religious persuasion, this might be expressed as
riving to live in harmony with the word and expectations of
od. For others, it might be expressed as focusing on living
harmony with the *Universe*.

hatever our belief and terminology, even as we become
less able" – or, at some stages, "differently able" – we still
rive to be as engaged as possible and to live in harmony
ith ourselves, our circumstances, our surroundings and
ith those around us. Even when these are not pleasant or
pretty" circumstances, we are most whole, most healthy,
hen we choose to embrace our situations rather than deny
em. This approach helps us live more fully.

olunteering is great for our communities and lso great for our own health, as well!
e enhance our quality of life by being as directly involved
s possible in those things that are nurturing to us, those
hings that bring us joy, those things that help us feel
aluable and needed.

here are many opportunities for being involved in our
ommunities. ***Being engaged in our own lives and the***
ives of our communities enhances our physical, emotional
nd spiritual well-being. It helps us feel a sense of
nterconnectedness with our communities (ideally, with all of
reation!), and it helps nurture a more fulfilling environment
n which we and our fellow community members can thrive.

olunteering and unselfishly doing good for others helps
s live more fully and positively and enhances our health
nd well-being. Studies of people age 60 and older who
ngage in volunteer work indicate that they describe
hemselves as feeling more physically active and energetic,
ess marginalized (that is, more directly involved, rather than

387

sitting on the sidelines), less sad or depressed, and happier and more hopeful for the future as a result of the social interactions.

In our RSVP program, we are told by our more than 1000 local "senior" volunteers that while they volunteer to "give back" to the community, not to receive any publicity or public thanks, nonetheless they also receive tremendous benefits . . . they feel involved, "still with it" and needed. Strong evidence exists that seniors who are involved in intergenerational activities – for example, tutors, mentors or others who work with children and young people – feel even more involved in their society . . . reflecting again a sense of interconnectedness.

As one of our 82-year-old volunteers recently exclaimed, "Knowing you're needed is a great feeling . . . the best, really! Everybody needs to feel needed!"

What other documentation exists for the claim that people who remain engaged in their communities enhance their health and well-being?

A recent **National Geographic** article, "The Secrets of Long Life" (November 2005), linked *community connectedness* to *longevity*. This reinforced what our volunteers have been telling us for years!

At our 2005 annual RSVP Volunteer Recognition event, we surveyed 442 senior volunteers. Over 95% of those volunteers said that volunteering helps to keep them physically and mentally active, and nearly all of them said that volunteering helps them to be connected to the community.

at prompted one of my RSVP colleagues, Program ordinator Dave Layton, to do additional research. "We alized that, between the records in our computer database d our ability to search for obituaries on the Internet, we ight be able to support or refute those volunteers' opinions ith statistics," Dave explained. "We decided it would be teresting to conduct a study comparing longevity of Quad ity RSVP members with the longevity of their peers in the neral population locally."

onnie Liedtke, one of our RSVP office volunteers from avenport, Iowa, graciously offered to help with this study y spending many hours searching through obituaries r former local RSVP members who had volunteered least 500 lifetime hours. Bonnie found obituaries of neral population members based on strict numerical and oportional demographic guidelines.

ur study indicated that the former RSVP members lived an verage of three years longer than their general population ers.

ave then submitted our results, methodology and raw data Professor Dan Corts of the Augustana College Psychology epartment, Rock Island, Illinois. He and Brett Wells, one f his students, reviewed our information and performed a tatistical analysis of our data using two different methods. heir findings were:

- that the "difference is statistically significant" when measuring the mean and standard deviation of the ages of the two groups.
- when measuring confidence intervals, "there is less than a 5% chance that the true population means are in the reverse order -- RSVP'ers achieving a lower age."

389

Professor Corts noted that although the sampling methods were not identical, "We would have a very high likelihood of getting similar results; that is, the RSVP mean would still be above the general population."

Although we were excited by this validation from a statistics expert, nonetheless, we understood early on that our RSVP sample was incomplete. We've only been keeping thorough computer records for 5 years. Some of our former members may have retired from volunteering before then and lived to a ripe old age. Others may have moved to parts unknown and we could not find their obituary. However, even with these disclaimers, it is clear that the average longevity of RSVP volunteers would probably be even longer if we had all the information.

So, Dave says, in a nutshell, we can now say, "Evidence shows that RSVP members who have volunteered over 500 lifetime hours live longer than their peers in the general population." It must be noted that this is a comparison with members of the general population, not necessarily only non-volunteers. Some of those people might actually volunteer on their own. Certainly if we compared volunteer longevity with non-volunteer longevity, the difference could be even more pronounced.

It's important to understand what this study says and what it doesn't say. It doesn't address whether volunteering makes people healthy or rather healthy people volunteer. It also doesn't address whether or not volunteering is just one facet of an overall healthier lifestyle which includes recreation, spirituality and family support.

So, even though this study does not prove that volunteering promotes longevity, when you combine it with the opinions those surveyed volunteers who believe it does promote ood health, it's safe to say, **"Volunteer! It's good for the ommunity and it's good for you!"**

What other benefits exist for senior volunteers?

addition to the satisfaction that comes from knowing ou've done a good job and made a difference in the life of our community, there are several other advantages to being volved with a Senior Corps program such as RSVP. Other enior Corps programs administered by the Corporation for ational Community Service (CNCS) include the Foster randparents Program (FGP) and the Senior Companion rogram (SCP).

Reimbursement for Transportation to Volunteer Work ssignments: RSVP offers senior volunteers the opportunity seek reimbursement for some of their mileage expenses curred in getting to and from their volunteer assignments. lthough usually reimbursed at a relatively low rate (e.g., 15 ents per mile for a maximum of $15 mileage reimbursement er month), this makes a big difference to some of our olunteers, who indicate that without the reimbursement, ney probably would not be able to afford to continue to olunteer.

Supplemental Insurance: While participating in ommunity service through RSVP, volunteers are covered t no cost by three kinds of insurance: accident, personal ability and excess automobile liability while volunteering r traveling to and from volunteering. This is considered econdary coverage, supplemental to the volunteer's primary uto insurance coverage.

Volunteer-recognition Activities: Active RSVP members /ho volunteer and report at least 12 hours of community

391

service through RSVP are invited to events at which their contributions to their respective communities are recognized. These events, co-sponsored by our RSVP Advisory Council and often attended by local, regional and national community leaders, are fun and always are well-attended.

"Safe living" / emergency-preparedness focus: Our local RSVP focuses on providing information and encouragement to seniors to be prepared for the possibility of personal or community emergency. We help seniors build emergency-preparedness plans, and we are actively involved in bi-state, interagency preparedness drills and simulations, in which we involved our volunteers, as well.

Active volunteers get noticed . . . when they're present, and when they're not! Many of us worry that we or our loved ones might become ill and that no one will know that we or they are ill until much later. One of the best "fringe benefits" about being actively involved in the community is that there are more people who are aware when you are present and when you are not. We frequently receive calls from volunteers, family members or administrators of community agencies where we place volunteers, indicating that they haven't seen a particular volunteer for a while and are concerned. That has been great comfort to volunteers and their families alike . . . an unofficial but very important fringe benefit of being actively involved in the community!

Getting connected to community resources for seniors: Our RSVP is sponsored by *Western Illinois Area Agency on Aging* (WIAAA), Rock Island, with offices at WIAAA in Rock Island and at *Generations Area Agency on Aging* in Davenport.

A wonderful network of 650 Area Agencies on Aging exists nation-wide to assist seniors in finding resources they need remain independent and safe in their homes for as long as possible.

The local Area Agencies on Aging are an excellent "first stop" when seeking information regarding resources for seniors and their caregivers:

- ***Western Illinois Area Agency on Aging*** *(Bureau, Henderson, Henry, Knox, LaSalle, McDonough, Mercer, Putnam, Rock Island, Warren counties, Illinois)* – 309.793.6800 / 800.322.1051, www.wiaaa.org.

- ***Generations Area Agency on Aging*** *(Scott, Clinton and Muscatine counties, Iowa)* 563.324.9085 / 800.892.9085; www.genage.org.

The WIAAA Website has excellent links to senior resources throughout the nation, which are helpful for seniors, caregivers, family members and other concerned persons: http://www.wiaaa.org/links/links.htm. I encourage you to check out the WIAAA Website – the ***"First Stop for Seniors"*** when looking for information.

In addition, ***United Way of the Quad Cities Area*** coordinates ***InfoLINK***, an excellent resource for matching individual and community needs and resources: 563.355.9900 or 888.680.4636 (www.unitedwayqc.org/infolink).

How can seniors become involved in volunteer work?

Churches, schools, libraries, museums, after-school programs, senior centers and many other community organizations often have roles for volunteers to play. Our communities are eager for the experience, knowledge, wisdom, skills and time which "seasoned" volunteers are able to offer.

If you are 55 years of age or older, feel free to call or email *"RSVP" -- the Retired and Senior Volunteer Program of Eastern Iowa & Western Illinois* (309.793.4425; shartung@wiaaa.org). This local RSVP is a program of the Corporation for National and Community Service (CNCS), with funding from the states of Iowa (Iowa Commission on Volunteer Service) and Illinois (Illinois Department on Aging), United Way of the Quad Cities Area, Riverboat Development Authority, and corporate and private donations

There are no restrictions based on income, race, education, experience, gender, disabling conditions, religion, national origin, employment history or political affiliation. We make a conscious effort to recruit volunteers who reflect the diversity and richness of our communities.

We'd be delighted to talk with you and share the hundreds of volunteer opportunities that are available at the more than 130 community organizations which we assist in securing volunteers.

Stay engaged and keep sharing your talents and spirit!

Remember: Stay positive, remain focused on what would help you enjoy your life and be fulfilled, continue bringing beauty into your life (work through the anger and "lose" negative people and situations when possible!) and let others know how they can help (you and their communities). Most of all, keep looking for the beauty in life, even as personal and health situations change.

It's ALL gift, even the challenges!

So . . . with this in mind . . . go forth, do good (and well!) and keep on engaging in gracious living and graceful aging!

394

bdomen   36, 37, 40, 58, 81, 339, 342, 346

bdominal pain   58, 59, 66

bdominoplasty   342

bnormalities   64, 118, 232, 233

ccidents   5, 9, 289, 351, 391

ctivities, sexual   257, 258, 274

cupuncture   192, 193

ge-related changes   266, 279

ging   vii, ix, xi, 1, 4-6, 8, 13, 24, 43, 49, 53, 102, 113, 253, 254, 338, 364, 365, 380, 381, 383-385, 392-394

lcohol   60, 62, 70, 72, 108, 111, 126, 141-143, 145, 160, 222, 228, 249, 263, 269

lignment   286, 292, 294, 301

lternative Medicine   187, 189, 199

lzheimer's disease   9, 43, 46-52, 143, 268, 287

merican Cancer Society   227, 238

msler grids   330

NA   247-249

neurysms   40, 41, 46

nger   123, 155, 157, 214, 236, 394

ngina   16, 76, 77

ngiogram   17, 18, 34, 37, 39

ngioplasty   15-18, 20, 37, 119

nkles   33, 34, 169, 179, 288, 297

nterior segment   323-325

ntibiotics   26, 113, 306, 309

ntibodies   241, 247, 248, 249, 307, 310

ntibody tests   248

ntidepressants   145, 156, 275-277, 325, 366

nti-inflammatory medications   303

nonsteroidal   281, 297

ntioxidants   48, 208, 209, 339

nxiety   52, 59, 61, 62, 123, 155, 157, 165, 231, 236, 258, 265, 279

Appetite   85, 88, 137, 138, 146, 271, 275, 279

ARBs   74, 76, 96

Arch   296, 297

Areolar   345

Arms   16, 34, 60, 67, 169, 179, 180, 282, 307, 310

Arteries   9, 15-20, 23, 29, 31, 32, 34-41, 43, 68-70, 75, 76, 115, 121, 143, 144, 254

   vertebral   37, 39

Arthritis   6, 33, 52, 169, 171, 184, 193, 210, 241, 244, 245, 247, 267, 268, 281, 283, 284, 297-300

Aspirin   17, 19, 46, 68, 145, 242, 309

Assets   352, 353, 361

Asymptomatic bacteriuria   312

Atherosclerosis   38, 69, 115, 254, 256

Attorney   352, 354, 360

Autoimmune diseases   241

B

Balance   7, 67, 81, 108, 109, 138, 151, 171-173, 175, 177, 178, 183, 195, 196, 202, 207, 219-221, 376

Ball   288, 292, 296, 300

Balloon   15, 18, 19, 35, 40

Bands   173, 178, 180, 296

Beans   93, 131, 135, 141, 143

Beliefs   163, 195, 198, 200, 387

Bereavement   272

Beta-blockers   74, 76

Beverages   132, 148, 155, 159, 162

Biopsy   25, 231

Blisters   311

Blockages   13, 15, 17-20, 22, 27, 29, 31-38, 70, 256

Blocked arteries, open   35

Blockers, beta   17, 22, 23, 28, 29

Blockers, calcium channel   17, 74, 77

Blood   14-18, 21, 22, 24, 26, 27, 29, 37, 38, 43, 74, 113, 139-141, 244, 253, 261, 262, 292, 330, 341, 342

clots   18, 36, 46, 51, 65, 67, 68, 110, 145, 290, 291

flow   31-33, 35, 39, 43, 44, 67, 116, 216

flows of   75, 76

pressure   7, 20, 23, 28, 29, 31, 34, 35, 56, 59, 70-72, 75-78, 96, 105, 114, 115, 142, 144, 145

medications   96, 221, 223

high   74

sugar readings   83, 84, 97

sugars   62, 63, 82, 83, 88, 90-93, 95-97, 115, 116, 119, 135, 139, 140, 171, 172, 183, 333, 334

fasting   82, 255

tests   27, 76, 83, 95, 231, 255

thinners   17, 25, 29, 68, 317

vessels   xi, 13-18, 20, 26-28, 31, 37, 43, 55, 64, 69, 77, 114-116, 121, 330, 332-335

BMI   154, 166, 167

Body   24, 27-29, 31, 32, 43-45, 62-67, 75-77, 81, 108, 109, 136, 138, 139, 145, 154-158, 172, 191-193, 206, 215, 216, 218-220, 225, 232-236, 306, 345

fat   154, 184

weight   41, 130, 154, 159, 285

healthy   132

ideal   30, 39, 244

lower   35

normal   73

Bone

density   106, 138

disease   111

formation   101, 102, 107, 111

fractures   101, 102, 106, 109-111, 297

health   101-103, 108, 109

loss   102-104, 107, 108, 127

mass   103, 106-109, 144, 184

scan   232

Bones   vii, 33, 101-104, 105, 107-111, 142, 154, 169, 208, 225, 232, 284, 289, 290, 293-297, 301, 364

Botox   338

Brain   16, 26, 37, 38, 40, 41, 43-53, 59, 64, 65, 67, 69, 77, 124, 26●, 268, 275, 277

Breads   91, 92, 109, 131, 134, 149

Breasts   144, 225, 226, 230, 343-34●

Breath   25, 57, 62, 63, 65, 123, 182, 216, 219

shortness of   14-16, 21, 22, 24, 25, 30, 55, 60, 61, 63-65, 169, 174●, 183, 309

Breathe   58, 122, 125, 178, 180, 18●

Breathing   10, 57, 58, 122, 124, 12●, 164, 216-219

BRM   244

Bruits   38, 39

Bump   297, 299, 300

Bunions   96, 297-301

Bursitis   250, 284

Byetta   88, 89

Bypass surgery   20, 119

C

Cabbage   143, 144

CAD   14, 32, 37, 39, 256

Caffeine   61, 62, 108, 126, 145, 161●, 202, 222

Calcium   27, 77, 101, 108, 109, 131, 138, 142, 143, 145, 165, 208

Calories   7, 92-94, 130-134, 138, 140, 150, 155, 156, 160, 165, 167, 172, 184

Canal, nerve   302, 303

Cancer   viii, xi, 8, 9, 11, 43, 102, 121, 129, 143, 144, 153, 154, 181, 195, 225-227, 229-241, 267, 268

breast   110, 225, 345

cells   225, 234, 235

diagnosis   229-231, 235, 238

information 237, 240
medications 229
patients 238
prevention 227, 239, 240
**Cancer Recovery Healthy
    Exchanges Cookbook** 228
Cancer, recurrences of 236, 237
Cancer Research 227, 228, 239
Cancer
  risk of 121, 144, 209
  treatments 102, 229
Cane 170, 184, 283, 285
Carbohydrates 81, 86, 91-94, 98,
    139, 140
Cardiac 20, 21
Cardiomyopathy 13, 21-23, 28, 29
Cardiovascular disease 69, 82, 115,
    127, 153, 256, 257
Caregivers 48, 270, 393
Carotid arteries 28, 31, 37-40, 46,
    114
Cartilage 286
Cataract surgery 316-318, 328
Cataracts 95, 315-318, 324, 325,
    333, 364
Catheter 34, 35, 39-41
Cells 81, 113, 136, 139, 208, 225,
    241, 244, 247, 248, 329, 379
Census 1-3, 6, 8
Challenges xi, 269, 270, 364, 366,
    367, 369, 378, 394
Charities 361
Cheese 63, 130, 131, 137, 140, 142
Chemicals 204, 208, 332
Chemotherapy 230, 234, 236, 237
Chest 16, 21, 30, 40, 55, 57, 60, 61,
    169, 178, 180
  pain 14-16, 25, 30, 32, 55, 56, 59-
    61, 64, 119, 174, 259
Chew 91, 126, 146, 147
Children 4, 49, 196, 205, 289, 294,
    296, 342, 352, 353, 368, 369,
    388
Chills 65, 66, 307
Chiropractors 189, 191, 192

Cholesterol vii, 15, 31, 34, 37, 39,
    105, 113-119, 130, 135, 140,
    141, 143, 171, 172
  bad 114-116, 118, 135, 140
  build-up of 38, 39
  good 114, 116, 118, 140
  levels 113, 116, 117, 119
Chondroitin 244, 245
Choroid 326, 330
Chronic Diseases 9, 199, 256, 306,
    332
Chronic Illness 129, 267
Cialis 56, 257-260
Cigarettes 34, 124-126
Claudication 31, 33, 35
Clinical trials 234, 235, 369-371
Coffee 133, 136, 162, 222
Colon 25, 121, 143, 144, 225, 230,
    232
Communities ix, xii, 279, 280, 363,
    383, 384, 387, 388, 391-394
Community foundation 361, 362
Comorbidities 8, 9
Complications 25, 56, 69, 105, 221,
    263, 266, 274, 293, 306, 308,
    311, 333, 371
Compressions 57
Conditions 13, 14, 25, 27-29, 47,
    50, 51, 58, 65, 66, 69-71, 81,
    96, 97, 193, 195, 274, 281, 282,
    297-299, 329, 330
Confusion 10, 30, 44, 61, 62, 66,
    67, 109, 196, 204, 209, 271
Consumption 72, 116
Contact 62, 64, 66-68, 181, 215,
    379, 381
Continuum 188, 221, 383-385
Controversy 195, 198, 208
Cool-down 177, 178
Coronaries 13, 17, 18
Coronary artery disease 14, 31, 32,
    39, 115, 117, 256
Cough 66, 121, 122, 307, 309
CPR 56, 58
CT scan 27, 34, 40, 45, 232, 285

Cures 51, 71, 188, 197, 290, 313, 325, 331, 369, 370
Cytokines 241, 244

D
DASH eating plan 72, 73, 137, 142
Death xi, 7, 9-11, 16, 20, 29, 30, 51, 68, 69, 101, 105, 114, 115, 306, 308-310, 353, 360, 361
Degenerative changes 13, 27, 30, 329, 331
Degree 28, 39, 115, 118, 148, 191, 194, 245, 246, 295, 345
Dehydrated patients 28
Dementia 46, 47, 50, 137, 143, 268, 272, 287
Depression xi, 21, 47, 48, 155, 157, 171, 236, 257, 265-280, 311
  diagnosis of 265, 273
  history of 267
  late-life 267
  prevention of 278, 279
  relapse of 277
  symptoms of 266, 269, 271, 273-279
Desserts 92, 146, 149, 151
Devices 61, 262, 303, 346, 351, 369-371
Diabetes xi, 6, 8, 9, 22, 23, 34, 35, 38, 39, 76, 81-89, 93-99, 139, 140, 143, 144, 153, 254-257, 267, 332-334
  medications 84, 89, 90, 91
  mellitus 8, 10
Diabetic
  neuropathy 96, 97
  retinopathy 95, 315, 332-334
Diabetics 16, 28, 62, 114, 115, 117, 181, 220, 333
Diagnosis 17, 32, 37, 47, 52, 233, 254, 271, 273, 274, 284, 322, 375
Diet 5, 7, 15, 73, 91-93, 97, 99, 107, 108, 114, 116, 135, 139, 141, 158, 159, 206-208, 222

  healthy 46, 48, 52, 111, 130, 166, 226, 227, 263, 275
  pills 166
  vegetarian 137, 164
Dietary Guidelines 129, 130, 137, 168
Disability 101, 119, 267
Disciplines 189, 192, 195, 352
Disease 43, 46, 47, 49, 51, 88, 89, 115, 142-144, 166, 182, 183, 188, 221, 309, 310, 317-320, 332, 333, 364, 365
Disease Control 8, 10, 11
Disease, infectious 306
Disease Modifying Drugs 243
Disease
  process 295, 369, 370
  risk 154, 155
  states 188
  symptoms 50
  transmitted 227, 312, 313
Distance 35, 178, 213, 316, 318
Distribution 1, 352, 353, 356, 358, 360
Disturbances, electrical 28-30, 77
Diuretics 23, 66, 74, 76, 249
Dizziness 27, 28, 44, 56, 59, 60, 61, 65, 67, 77, 78, 169, 174, 177, 260, 276
Doctor ix, 59-62, 66-68, 116-119, 230-232, 234, 254, 256-259, 263, 276, 283-285, 317, 318, 347, 348, 370-373, 375-378
Documents 288, 352, 353, 380
Dose 51, 56, 73, 85, 117, 197, 258, 260, 310, 370
Drink 52, 62, 63, 70, 73, 91, 94, 97, 109, 136, 145, 147, 148, 161, 222, 226, 228
Drinking 62, 82, 136, 138, 144
Driving ix, 16, 55, 181, 183, 317, 363-368
Drug interaction 78, 117

Drugs 23, 29, 74, 75, 78, 85, 86, 117-119, 145, 196, 197, 234, 235, 242, 243, 246, 258, 259, 261, 365, 366, 370, 371
  disease-modifying 243
  experimental 246, 370
  life-saving 113
DXA 106, 107, 111

E

Eating 36, 37, 59, 60, 62, 63, 82, 84, 85, 88, 111, 135-137, 140, 143-145, 147, 148, 155-158, 161-166, 274, 305, 306
  calcium-rich foods 142
  healthy 41, 127, 151
Effectiveness 75, 80, 189, 198, 240, 246, 276, 277, 322, 370
Electrolytes 27, 62, 63, 66, 97
Emergency vii, 55, 60, 61, 65, 349, 379-381
Emotional hunger 157, 158
Endurance 170, 173, 177, 178, 180, 287, 290
Energy 81, 92, 93, 122, 131, 132, 139, 156, 161, 171, 192, 212-215, 218, 219, 223, 234, 271
Epidemiology vii, 1
Erectile dysfunction viii, 56, 253, 257, 262
Erection 253, 254, 258, 259, 261, 262
Estate 351-353, 359-362
Ethnicity 2, 3
Evaluation 30, 60, 71, 75, 101, 248, 255, 264, 284, 316, 320, 321
Exercise viii, 7, 15, 23, 30, 41, 52, 53, 89, 90, 126, 127, 132, 133, 155, 156, 169-172, 174-177, 180-183, 287, 288
  endurance 179
  heart rates 182, 183
  program 20, 109, 169, 173, 176, 177, 285, 287

  regular 39, 46, 49, 109, 166, 222, 270
  routines 178, 183
Experience 16, 20, 27, 30, 37, 55, 58, 60, 61, 63-65, 191, 192, 215, 267-269, 271-273, 333, 393, 394
  symptoms 271, 302
Exubera 87, 88
Eye 64, 69, 84, 95, 216, 241, 315-319, 321-324, 326, 328, 332, 333, 335, 337, 338, 340, 364, 365
  pressure 322, 323, 333

F

Factors 39, 104, 107, 111, 115, 155, 200-202, 229, 266, 302, 316, 321, 322, 337, 347, 355
Fainting 25-30, 59, 61, 65, 67
Families 209, 238, 351, 381, 392
Fat 93, 94, 132, 139, 141, 146, 150, 154, 155, 159, 166, 172, 207, 227, 337, 338, 340-343
  saturated 116, 130, 140, 141, 159, 227
  trans 116, 130, 141, 159
Fatigue 14, 62, 65, 71, 76, 123, 157, 169, 171, 236, 265, 271, 296
Feelings 28, 61, 65, 96, 123, 126, 129, 155, 157, 158, 161, 171, 236, 265, 271-274, 387, 388
Feet 28, 34, 35, 96, 97, 248, 249, 295, 296, 299-301, 338, 364
  flat 295, 296
Females 1, 4, 6, 16, 86, 134, 153, 154, 298
Fever 64-66, 256, 305-307, 309, 310, 312
Fiber 30, 59, 93, 131, 132, 135, 136, 139, 147, 160, 164
Fibromyalgia 249, 250, 379
Fight xi, 141, 156, 171, 216, 235, 279

File of life pouches 380
Financial advisor 354, 355, 357, 358, 362
Fish 48, 131, 133, 145, 148, 150, 207, 227
  cold-water 140, 144
  oils 109, 118, 140, 206, 207, 222, 245
Fitness Benefits 173, 174, 182
Flashes 326, 328
Flatfoot 295-297
Flexibility 139, 172, 173, 175-178, 184, 218, 219, 303, 364, 366
Floaters 326, 333, 334
Flows 212, 213, 219, 322, 383
Flu 63, 97, 256, 305-310
Fluids 8, 22, 59, 97, 136, 147, 192, 233, 320-323, 328, 330
Folds 256, 337, 338, 381
Foods 37, 58, 60, 62, 81, 86-88, 92-94, 108-110, 129-132, 135-143, 145-151, 155, 157-160, 164-166, 227, 228, 306
Foot 33, 96, 97, 295-298, 300, 301
Footwear 170, 296, 300, 301
Forget 47, 92-94, 364, 368
Foundation xi, xii
Fractures vii, 101, 103-105, 107, 108, 110, 138, 142, 288, 291-295
Fruit juice 91, 130, 131, 141, 160
Fruits 30, 73, 92, 116, 130, 131, 133, 135, 139, 141, 143, 148, 149, 151, 160, 228
  citrus 135, 144, 147
  dried 130, 131, 133, 145

G
Genetics 6, 15, 92, 107, 108, 299
Glaucoma 95, 315, 318-323, 325, 333, 364
  narrow angle 323-325
  open angle 319, 320, 322, 323, 325
Glucosamine 244, 245

Glucose 81, 82, 85, 86, 88, 92, 139
  tablets 87, 91, 92
Goal setting 158, 159
Goals 20, 35, 89, 158, 159, 163, 164, 172, 175-177, 179, 189, 214, 215, 219, 221, 223, 224, 230, 235
  long-term 126, 161, 164
Gout 154, 249
Grains 92, 116, 130, 131, 133, 135, 139, 143, 144, 160, 227
Grapefruit juice 78-80
Grief 272
Groin 18, 36, 39-41, 58
Growth 1, 3, 25, 226, 234, 260, 341, 355, 357, 361

H
Hahnemann 196-198
Hallucinations 272, 273, 275
Hallux 297, 298, 299, 300
Harmony 385-387
HDL 113, 114, 116-118, 140
Head 25, 31, 37, 38, 57, 63, 64, 157, 158, 178, 272, 282, 294
Headaches 38, 43, 56, 63, 64, 192, 259, 260, 307, 323
Heal 115, 188, 191, 213, 226, 290, 292, 305
Healing 10, 188, 193, 195-197, 212, 213, 217, 218, 301, 323
  secrets 199
Health 6, 7, 10, 11, 82, 83, 91, 94, 95, 97, 98, 101, 136-139, 191, 192, 223, 224, 228, 229, 236-238, 375, 379, 386-388
  benefits 171, 172, 174, 182, 212, 287
  conditions 69, 125, 378
    chronic 6, 8, 139
  declining 269
  history, personal 209
  program 219, 220
  providers 210
  risks 127, 153

Health Statistics 8, 10, 11
Healthcare provider 97, 200, 254, 269, 273-277, 280
Healthy eating plan 142
Heart xi, 13-27, 29-31, 35-37, 43, 46, 52, 55, 61, 62, 68, 69, 75-77, 83, 84, 121, 122, 168, 169, 233
  arteries 20
  attack 13-17, 20, 21, 32, 55, 68, 74, 77, 82, 114, 115, 117, 142, 144, 169, 267, 268
  beats 27, 30, 76
    irregular 29, 30, 169
  blood vessels 18
  disease vii, 6, 8, 9, 13-15, 20, 69, 93, 96, 113-115, 121, 133, 139, 141, 143, 144, 153
    accounts 30
    coronary 46
    developing 116
    fighting 30
    progression 30
    risk of 135, 144
  failure 13, 14, 21-23, 25, 65, 66, 70, 71, 76, 86, 114, 142
    congestive 9, 20, 22, 25, 76
  health 105, 135
  muscle 14-16, 18, 20-22, 27, 29, 30, 55, 76, 77, 116
    problem, intrinsic 21
    stiff 23
    weak 13, 23, 28, 29
  rate 28, 76, 77, 182, 183, 216
  rhythm 16, 20, 27-29, 119, 208
  rhythms, abnormal 27, 29, 61, 62
  strength 23
  valves 13, 24, 25, 29
    abnormal 25, 26
Heartbeat, irregular 9, 67, 71
Heartburn 59, 60, 147, 236
Heel 57, 295, 296
Heirs 352, 360, 361
Herbal
  medicines 199, 201, 202, 204, 205

  remedies 199-201, 204, 221, 229, 277
Herbs 142, 146, 150, 200, 202-205, 229, 269
HF 22, 23
High blood pressure 9, 22, 23, 30, 32, 38, 39, 41, 46, 59, 66, 67, 69-71, 74, 76-78, 80, 142, 153
Hip 33, 103, 105, 249, 288-292, 295, 302
  fractures 103, 105, 288-290
  replacement 292
    minimally-invasive 292, 293
Hispanic 2, 3, 83
History 17, 20, 23, 32, 38, 49, 70, 221, 227, 250, 267, 269, 296, 299, 308
HIV 312, 313
Holes 102, 326, 328
Home 11, 20, 60, 83, 97, 105, 109, 123, 151, 181, 234, 236, 269, 292, 347-349
  health aide 348
Homeopathy 196, 198, 199
Hormones 79, 88, 139, 234, 235, 257, 266
Hospital ix, 11, 16, 17, 20, 55, 63, 234, 238, 328, 347, 349, 368, 371
Hours 15, 17, 26, 27, 34, 45, 58, 60, 63, 66, 82, 87, 97-99, 149, 158, 258-260
  lifetime 389, 390
Human body 92, 370
Humerus 282
Hunger 62, 82, 90, 157, 158, 161, 162, 279
Hurt 108, 212, 297, 299, 301
Hypertension 6-8, 13, 15, 23, 69-72, 74, 77, 80, 131, 142-144, 217, 221, 256, 257, 379
Hypoglycemia 62, 90

I
Ill 97, 98, 170, 392

Illnesses 6, 63, 82, 97, 98, 129, 148, 171, 245, 248, 250, 266, 267, 272, 274, 279, 309
  life-threatening 267, 268, 271
Images 34, 232, 233
Imaging, magnetic resonance 45, 232
Imbalance 26, 27, 195, 220
  chemical 266, 268
Immune system 148, 210, 229, 235, 241, 243, 244, 305
Implant 345, 346
Impotence 253, 254, 264
Inability 6, 16, 22, 67, 107, 123, 171, 253, 270-272, 274
Income 348, 358, 361, 394
Independence xii, 101, 108, 171, 274, 278, 363
Index, body mass 73, 154, 166
Indicators 210, 211, 256
Infections ix, xi, 9, 20, 21, 25, 26, 43, 45, 51, 148, 207, 209, 241, 261, 305, 306, 309
Infiltrative diseases 22, 23
Inflammation 21, 184, 191, 194, 206, 207, 241-244, 281, 285
Inflammatory rheumatic diseases 241, 243
Influenza 9, 10, 65, 305-307
Information 71, 74, 161, 163, 194, 200, 201, 210, 211, 224, 238-240, 284, 335, 375-378, 380, 381, 389, 390, 392, 393
  sheets 380, 381
    personalized 379
Ingredients, active 199, 201, 202, 205
Injections 13, 82, 87, 88, 234, 261, 281, 283, 285, 310, 331, 332, 338
  corticosteroid 282
Injury 108, 178, 180, 191, 219, 262, 284, 287, 288, 295, 351
Insulin 62, 63, 81-83, 85-89, 97, 139, 220

  medication stimulates 85
Insulin Secretagogue 85
Insurance 359, 371, 378, 381, 391
Intake 62, 130, 141, 144, 222
Integrative Medicine 187-189
Integrity 294, 383, 385, 386
Intensity 28, 58, 170, 174-176, 184, 185
Interest 200, 201, 219, 223, 278
Intraocular pressure 321, 325, 333
Iris 323, 326, 333
Ischemic stroke 43, 45, 46

J
Januvia 89
Jaw line 337, 339
Joints 33, 133, 136, 170, 171, 184, 241, 242, 244, 247, 249, 284, 287, 288, 302, 364

K
Ketoacidosis 63
Kidney disease 9, 70, 89, 102, 95, 96
Kidneys 31, 52, 65, 66, 69, 70, 75, 84-86, 95, 96, 116, 136, 140, 233, 248, 267
Knee 33, 244, 249, 283, 285, 286, 302
  replacement 283, 284, 286
    surgery 283
    total 285-287

L
Laser 193, 322, 328, 331, 334, 341
LDL 113-116, 118, 140
  cholesterol 135, 141, 143, 144
L-dopa 50
Leak 13, 23-25, 29
Legacy 359, 361, 362
Legal advisor 352, 354
Legs 20, 31-37, 49, 66, 67, 116, 169, 173, 179, 180, 296, 302, 341, 364
Lens 315-318, 324, 328, 333

Levitra 56, 257-260
Lewy Body Disease 51
Licensed dietitians 166, 167
Life
  expectancy 4-6, 10, 25, 113
  file of 380
  healthier 129
  healthy 81, 172
  insurance 359, 361
    contracts 359, 362
  last days of 10, 11
  span 4, 5
Lifeline 348, 349
Lifestyle viii, 5, 6, 82, 84, 134, 175,
    220, 227, 230, 265, 269
  changes 6, 15, 93, 158, 166, 167,
    235, 268, 278
  choices 5, 107
  healthy 72, 92, 99, 101, 127, 205,
    228, 390
  modifications 71, 72, 80, 114, 119
  unhealthy 205
Lift 180, 182, 345
Light 63, 134, 170, 174, 177, 179,
    180, 182, 184, 214, 290, 323,
    326, 332, 364
Liposuction 342, 343
List 79, 84, 123, 150, 181, 189, 206,
    226, 230, 231, 238, 325, 349,
    359, 375, 377, 378, 379
Liver 52, 75, 85, 86, 88, 116, 117,
    145, 225, 229
Living, graceful 383, 385, 386
Longevity 113, 388-390
Lose weight 92, 132, 133, 135, 141,
    142, 156, 164, 179
Losing muscle 132
Loss 67, 69, 101, 105, 108, 123,
    146, 265, 269, 272, 278, 319,
    330, 337, 344
Lovastatin, lipid-lowering
    medications 78
Love 278, 339, 342, 384

Low blood sugar 45, 59, 62, 83,
    85-88, 90-92
Lung disease xi, 122
Lungs 22, 52, 88, 122, 144, 148,
    168, 225, 230, 232, 241, 248,
    267, 309
Lupus 241, 243, 248, 249

M
Macula 329-331, 334
Macular degeneration
  age-related 328-330
  wet 329, 331, 332
Magnesium 131, 132, 208, 222
Males 1, 4, 6, 8, 83, 134, 153, 154,
    253, 257, 343
Manipulation 191, 195
Market 242, 258, 370, 371
Massage Therapy 193-196
MD vii-ix, xii, 13, 31, 43, 113, 228,
    253, 281, 305, 315, 337
Meal service 348, 349
Meals 60, 62, 83, 85-88, 133, 139,
    145-147, 149-151, 159, 160,
    163, 236, 269, 349
Meat 7, 92, 93, 131, 139, 227
Medical 83, 348, 349, 352, 381
  attention xii, 16, 55, 58-60, 64-66,
    68
  conditions 6, 28, 30, 102, 104,
    107, 156, 183, 205
  equipment 347, 348
  treatment 22, 25, 80, 257
Medicare 99, 308, 318, 347-349
Medication effects 50, 52
Medication Interaction 79, 269
Medication levels 78
Medication Magnitude 79
Medication
  problems 47
  reaction 147
  side effects 268
  therapy 277
  treatment 111

Medications 28-30, 50, 51, 74-78, 82-90, 108-110, 117-119, 182, 183, 200, 201, 220-223, 229, 259-263, 268, 269, 275-277, 325, 365, 366

Medications Amiodarone 79

Medications
   antihypertensive 74
   cardiac 28
   cases 62
   cause 77
   common 50, 285
   corticosteroid 281
   effective 77, 111
   experimental 246
   generic 75
   gout 145
   inject therapeutic 233
   mixing 118
   multiple 51, 91
   non-essential 51
   non-estrogen 110
   oral 97
   over-the-counter 268, 269, 276, 277
     pain 378
   prescribe 365
   prescribed 275
   prescription 102, 166, 201, 254, 271, 276
   prescriptions 166
   safe 325
   side effect 255
   sinus 325
   thyroid 102
   traditional 249
   work 137

Medicines viii, 1, 15, 18, 46, 48, 52, 55, 56, 67, 68, 187, 199, 200, 220-222, 260, 261, 310, 311, 369

Meditation 192, 215, 217-219

Members 11, 49, 99, 127, 196, 209, 229, 231, 237, 258, 269, 271, 278, 389, 390, 392, 393

Memory 43, 46-48, 67, 268, 272

Menopause 102, 103, 107, 108, 142, 156, 157, 289

Meridians 192

Metformin 85, 86, 97

Midfoot 295, 296

Midwest Cardiovascular Research Foundation xi, xii

Milk 63, 87, 91, 92, 94, 130, 131, 136, 139, 142, 147, 149, 162

Mimic stroke symptoms 45

Mind xi, xii, 5, 75, 157, 194, 206, 218, 219, 265, 266, 276, 379, 394

Minor risk factors 15

Minutes 16, 29, 35, 44, 52, 56, 64, 71, 73, 88, 89, 91, 160, 161, 172, 173, 177-179, 261, 262
   few 16, 28, 60, 174, 177, 182, 185, 302

Mitral 24, 25

MmHg 70, 73

Money 123, 166, 216, 352-355, 361

Monitor 23, 27, 30, 34, 58, 62, 66, 71, 80, 97, 140, 222, 235, 277

Mood, depressed 265

Mouth 57, 60, 78, 94, 127, 147, 148, 232, 337, 338

Movement 49, 57, 58, 101, 185, 191, 195, 328

MRI 27, 45, 232, 282, 285

MS vii, ix, xii, 13, 363

Muscle
   aches 307, 308, 310
   groups 178, 180
     large 173, 178, 179

Muscles 7, 13, 16, 23, 27, 77, 154, 170-172, 177-180, 193, 249, 250, 284, 285, 295, 296, 342, 364
   abdominal 343
   facial 338

Muscular dystrophy 49

Myofascial pain 250

ame 75, 87, 114, 192, 295, 312, 353, 372, 378, 379

arrowing 13, 16, 23, 24, 27, 29, 37, 39, 302, 325

ausea 28, 55, 60, 63, 86, 88, 89, 97, 146, 205, 230, 236, 260

eck 16, 28, 31, 37-40, 46, 60, 61, 64, 66, 126, 140, 169, 179, 249, 337, 339

eedles 193, 225, 233

erves 77, 250, 303, 310, 311

europathy 96

eurotransmitters 266, 275

icotine 123, 124, 127

ipple 57, 344-346

itro 55, 56

onsteroidal antiinflammatory drugs 242

ose 57, 146, 232, 301, 337, 338

RP 124, 125

SAIDs 242, 285, 286

ucleus 247, 248

umbness 33, 43, 44, 66, 67

utrients 52, 93, 132, 136, 143, 167, 206, 216

utrition viii, 101, 129, 133, 138, 158, 159, 239, 305

utritional supplements 138, 228, 229, 263

uts 93, 131, 132, 135, 140, 141, 143, 144, 159, 164, 228

bese 6, 8, 133, 153-155, 160

besity viii, 15, 32, 92, 93, 114, 129, 153, 155, 156, 167, 168, 172, 257, 287, 296

bituaries 389, 390

bservation 234, 235

CN viii, 225

ffice 21, 71, 95, 206, 234, 255, 262, 308, 317, 318, 334, 346, 378, 392

Omega-3 fatty acids 118, 140-142, 144, 165, 207, 245

Omega-6 207

Open-heart surgery 267

Operation 234, 342, 344, 346

Ophthalmologist 95, 316-318, 320, 321, 324-326, 328-330, 333-335

Optic nerve 318, 319, 321, 322, 326

Order 62, 71, 75, 81, 91, 114, 151, 156-158, 164, 172, 188, 189, 197, 225, 338, 348

Organs 25, 29, 31, 43, 52, 56, 96, 101, 116, 136, 156, 192, 197, 198, 215, 225

Orthopedist 284, 285, 287, 296, 298, 300, 304

Osteoarthritis 133, 154, 241, 242, 244, 245, 247, 364

Osteopenia 107

Osteoporosis vii, 101-108, 110, 111, 142, 171, 184, 208, 287, 289
    developing 104, 109, 111
    development of 102, 107, 108
    primary 102
    risk of 110, 208
    secondary 102

Outpatient procedure/surgery 317, 326

Over-the-counter 124, 276, 303

Overweight 6, 70, 83, 133, 153, 154, 160, 165, 169, 222, 244

Oxygen 16, 17, 55, 56, 216, 326

Oz 73, 91, 130-132, 162, 228, 377

P

Pain 17, 32, 33, 36-38, 55, 58, 60, 63-65, 182, 184, 185, 249, 250, 281-285, 291, 292, 295-297, 299-302, 310-312
    medications 193
    symptoms 295

Pain-free 11, 297, 300

Palpitation 61, 62

Pancreas 81, 230
Parkinson's disease 9, 49-52, 268, 325
Partners 223, 261-263, 313, 381
Patient 71, 223, 240, 274
Patients 15-23, 27-29, 31-33, 39, 40, 45, 47, 50, 68-72, 76, 187-189, 191, 244-250, 253, 254, 261, 262, 281-283, 285-287, 290-293, 319, 320-322, 330, 331-333, 339, 343, 344-347, 248, 377-379
Pelvis 288
Penile implants 262, 263
Penis 253-255, 258, 261, 262
Pericarditis 21
Personality 266, 271, 272
  changes 43, 47, 62
Pharmaceuticals 200, 201, 204, 211, 220, 332
Phase 20, 21, 370, 371
Phosphorus 101, 108, 138, 143
Physical
  activity 5, 6, 15, 92, 101, 107, 108, 134, 141, 158, 160-163, 169, 171, 172, 178, 219, 267, 269
  illness 266, 271, 273
  therapy 46, 50, 110, 250, 282, 289, 297, 303, 347, 348
Physician 25-27, 51, 52, 75, 166, 167, 169, 174, 182, 183, 188, 200, 201, 204, 205, 211, 212, 220, 221, 223, 226, 229, 230
Phytochemicals 135, 141, 143
Pills 56, 257-259
Placebo 246, 371
Plan 89, 119, 126, 127, 149, 170, 188, 222, 351, 352, 354-356, 358, 361, 370, 375, 380, 381
  qualified 359-361
Planning, financial ix, 351
Plants 143, 199, 201, 202, 204
Plavix 17, 46, 68
Pneumococcal disease 309, 310

Pneumonia 9, 10, 51, 65, 241, 271, 305-307, 309
Population 1-8, 29, 49, 69, 113, 199, 208, 288, 298, 299, 319, 389, 390
Position 28, 33, 57, 59, 77, 78, 180, 219, 345
Posterior segments 321, 323, 326
Post-herpetic neuralgia 311
Potencies 198, 204
Poultry 131, 133, 145, 148, 150, 227
Practitioner 191, 197, 198, 212-215, 219
Pre-diabetes 82
Preferences 11, 381
Prescription 124, 183, 247, 268, 269, 276, 303
Pressure 22, 25, 55, 60, 193-195, 321-323, 326, 364
  normal blood 70
Prevention 20, 48, 95, 110, 143, 237, 239, 240, 274, 278, 290, 309, 313
Principles 72, 191, 214, 217, 383
Products 149, 204, 206, 229, 370
  nicotine replacement 123-125
Progress 48, 51, 69, 96, 159, 162, 168, 173, 174, 176, 267, 277
Prostheses, penile 257, 262, 263
Protection 119, 307, 309, 310
Protein 23, 47, 93, 131, 132, 138, 164, 227, 249
Providers 80, 89, 91, 95, 97, 98, 101, 114, 136, 182, 183, 209, 210, 269, 274, 277, 348, 349, 379
Purity 204, 210, 211
PVD 31-34, 39

Q
Qi 192
Quitting 121, 122, 124, 125, 126, 165

noking   vii, 30, 32, 121, 122, 165, 331

aces   2, 3, 103, 394
adicals, free   208, 209, 339
ash   68, 75, 311, 343
ate   3, 5, 6, 30, 50, 83, 87, 88, 95, 101, 102, 105, 115, 142, 156, 174, 270
mortality   3, 4
ealAge   6
ecovery   238, 267, 272, 273, 297, 346
ecurrent strokes   46
ed   248, 333, 378, 380, 381
rice yeast extract   118
edness   241, 242, 308, 310, 325
eflexes   364-366
efrigerators   87, 148, 149, 380
eiki   195, 212-215, 219
practitioner   213-215
treatments   213, 215
elationship, physician-patient   223
elaxation   65, 126, 164, 213, 218
response   216, 217
esearch   ix, 78, 111, 144, 217, 228, 229, 235, 239, 240, 250, 293, 339, 369, 371-373, 389
esisting body weight   173
esources   94, 200, 205, 236, 238, 267, 392, 393
esults   7, 74-78, 104-107, 147, 148, 154-156, 165, 166, 169, 170, 195, 196, 244-246, 269, 270, 272, 273, 302, 311, 320, 321, 365, 366
etina   326, 328, 329, 332-334
etinal detachments   315, 326-328, 334
etinopathy   95, 332, 334
etirement   269, 270, 278, 351-358, 359, 361
heumatoid arthritis   102, 241-245, 247, 296

Rheumatologist   248, 251, 284
Risk   49, 91, 92, 96, 103-107, 109-111, 114, 115, 118, 119, 121, 143, 144, 153, 154, 166, 167, 255, 256, 266, 267, 307, 308, 324, 325
factors   14, 15, 23, 32, 34, 37, 39, 46, 49, 83, 107, 114, 115, 166, 255, 256, 319, 328, 329
high   14, 96, 110, 268-270
increased   86, 90, 108-110, 157
Roizen   6, 376, 377
Rotator cuff   281, 282
RSVP   382, 384, 389-392, 394
Rupture   13, 18, 40

S
Sag   340, 344, 345
Saliva   64, 136, 146-148
Salt   108, 126, 130, 142, 146, 150, 228
Scan, painless heart   232
Scapula   281, 282
Scars   292, 344, 345
Scleroderma   248
Screws   291, 292, 303
Secrets   156, 199
Seeds   93, 131, 132, 135, 141, 143, 164, 384
Self-healing ability   196
Senior volunteers   384, 388, 391
Seniors   xi, xii, 16, 308, 309, 312, 337, 363, 367, 380, 383-385, 388, 392, 393
Services   237, 240, 348, 349, 363, 384, 392
Servings   131, 132, 137, 144, 227
Shammas   vii, xii, 13
Shingles   305, 310-312
Shoes   96, 97, 295, 297-300
Shot   307, 308, 310
Shoulders   60, 105, 179, 180, 249, 250, 281-283
Shriveled Vitreous Body   327

Side effects 50, 56, 75, 77, 84, 85, 88, 89, 198, 199, 204, 205, 220, 230, 258, 260, 261, 268, 269, 276, 277, 365, 366

Signs 10, 25, 31, 45, 55, 57, 63, 83, 94, 105, 106, 226, 256, 271, 283, 337, 338

Skin 10, 33, 76, 144, 208, 226, 241, 247, 294, 305, 310, 311, 337-340, 343, 344, 346

cancer 208, 340

Smell 121, 123, 124, 146, 148

Smoke 41, 88, 104, 109, 121-127, 169, 222, 226, 342

Smoking 5, 32, 39, 62, 87, 109, 121-123, 125, 127, 165, 230, 247, 254, 255, 257, 337

Social worker 237, 348, 349

Society xi, 155, 206, 208, 209, 319, 375, 383, 388

Sodium 23, 70, 73, 97, 142, 143, 150, 155

Soluble fiber 135, 141

Soup 134, 147, 150

SPF 226, 339, 340

Spices 142, 146, 150

Spine 37, 284, 295, 302, 303

fractures 105, 110

Stairs 161, 169, 171, 179, 181, 283, 295

State income taxes 360, 361

States, static 383, 385

Statins 79, 117, 118

Stenosis, spinal 302, 303

Stents 15, 18, 19, 35, 37, 40, 68

Strength 49, 124, 125, 172, 173, 175, 177-179, 184, 211, 215, 219, 289-291, 303

Stress 5, 15, 18, 24, 25, 30, 61, 64, 114, 123, 126, 155, 157, 164, 215, 216, 270

test 17, 18, 27, 222

Stretch 173, 178, 184

Stretching 15, 18, 21, 28, 126, 173, 178, 179, 250, 300

Stroke 9, 20, 25, 27, 29, 31, 32, 38, 40, 43-46, 65, 67, 74, 114, 11., 117, 142-144, 153

multiple 47, 50

patients 268

risk 121

Students xi, 212-214, 218, 389

Substance abuse 217, 269, 273

Substances 115, 143, 196-198, 24.

Sugar 81, 88, 91, 126, 130-132, 139, 149, 155, 160, 161, 227

Suicide 9, 270, 271, 273

Sun exposure 109, 201, 337, 340

Sunscreens 208, 339

Supplements 118, 137, 138, 143, 145, 165, 205-212, 222, 229, 245-247

dietary 135, 210, 211

mineral 136, 228

over-the-counter 245

Support network 237, 238

Surgeon 40, 230, 292, 293, 303, 318, 322, 323, 335, 340, 342

orthopedic 284, 290, 292

plastic ix, 337, 338, 340

Surgery 20, 21, 35, 40, 41, 167, 234, 236, 237, 283-285, 289-292, 297, 300, 301, 316, 317, 318, 322, 323, 328, 337-339, 342-344

laser 318, 322, 331

trabeculectomy 322

Surgical treatment 285, 290, 301, 303

Sweating 55, 60, 62, 90

Swelling 14, 22, 36, 75, 169, 191, 241, 242, 295, 301, 308, 311, 334

Symbols 213, 214

Symlin 88, 89

Symptoms 15, 30-33, 43-45, 49-51, 55, 58-68, 82, 90, 91, 104, 123, 196, 197, 265, 271-273, 283, 284, 302, 303, 305

common 31, 312, 316

System 123, 196, 212, 219, 367, 375, 380
  drainage 322, 325, 326
  electrical 13, 26, 29, 30
  nervous 26, 27, 193, 195, 233, 250, 260

T
Table vii, 2, 3, 161, 162, 203, 204
Tablets 56, 75, 85
Taste 124, 146, 148
Tax advisor 352, 353, 355, 358
Taxes 352-354, 356, 360
Teachers 212, 214, 219
Team 167, 224, 229, 236, 237
Techniques 69, 125, 164, 191-194, 292, 293, 328, 345, 346
  minimally-invasive 40, 293
Tendonitis 250, 282, 284
Tendons 250, 251, 293, 295, 296, 299, 301
Testing blood sugars 83
Tests 27, 28, 34, 39, 45, 83, 84, 86, 95, 117, 196, 225, 231-233, 247, 248, 255, 367, 370-372
Therapies 23, 35, 71, 110, 187, 189, 190, 192, 193, 215, 217, 219, 235, 264, 277, 347
  antiresorptive 110
  complementary 187, 189, 220, 224
  hormone 234
  mind-body 217, 221
  radiation 234, 237, 255
  self-injection 257, 261, 262
Thighbone 288, 290, 292
TIA 39, 45
Tingling 34, 66, 67, 96, 213, 215
Tissues 31, 191, 225, 232, 234, 241, 332, 337, 346
Tobacco 107, 108, 111, 123, 124, 125, 126, 127
Toes 96, 294-299
Tone 26-28, 343
Tongue 56

Total body water 136
Touch 58, 194, 195, 237, 354, 368
TPA 45
Treatment options 230, 234, 235, 262, 297, 328, 331, 334
Trial 235, 277, 370-372
Triglycerides 15, 114, 116, 118, 141
Trust 353, 354, 361, 362
Trustee 353
Tummy tucks 342
Tumor 21, 195, 225, 233, 234, 295
  cancerous 225
  markers 231
Twins 247

U
United States 1, 9, 14, 20, 46, 49, 69, 113, 114, 143, 153, 171, 187, 253, 309, 319
Urinary tract infections 65, 305, 312
Urine 66, 139, 233, 249, 312

V
Vaccination 307, 309, 310
Vaccines 113, 306-310
Valves 13, 23-25, 27
Vascular disease, peripheral vii, 9, 31, 32, 39, 121, 256
  reconstructive surgery 257, 263
Vegetables 7, 30, 48, 53, 73, 92, 93, 109, 116, 130, 131, 133-135, 139, 141-143, 148, 150, 151, 227, 228
Veins 20, 36, 43, 234, 254, 341
Very effective medications 35, 110
Vessels 18, 24, 74, 116, 256, 331, 341
Viagra 56, 253, 257-260
Viruses 311, 143, 308
Vision 64, 104, 108, 316-318, 320, 328-334, 365
  loss 44, 139, 315, 328, 329, 331-334

Vitamins 5, 93, 102, 108, 109, 118, 132, 136-138, 143-145, 164, 208, 209, 229, 263, 269, 331, 339

Vocabulary 383-385

Volunteering 383, 387, 390, 391

Volunteers 384, 388-393

Vomiting 55, 59, 63, 64, 89, 97, 98, 136, 146

W

Walls 18, 77, 210, 326, 330, 333

Warmth 213, 241, 242

Warm-up 177, 178

Water 58, 59, 97, 134, 136, 145, 154, 170, 173, 184, 202, 218

Weakness 14, 22, 25, 43, 44, 61, 67, 90, 146, 302

Wear 171, 283, 298-300

Weight 33, 82, 84, 86, 127, 129, 140, 141, 153, 154, 156, 161, 163, 165, 167, 173, 180

  gain 86, 127, 156, 158, 165, 172, 337

  healthy 154, 226, 228

  loss 41, 82, 88, 89, 116, 138, 141, 155, 158, 160, 165-167, 244, 269, 273

Well-being ix, 83, 156, 218, 382, 383, 386-388

Women 23, 52, 69, 70, 73, 102, 103, 107, 108, 110, 113, 135, 141, 142, 156, 164, 165, 199, 289, 343-346

Workout 175, 176, 178, 184

Wrinkles 337-340

Wrist 101, 105, 179, 293, 295

X

X-rays 246, 281-283, 286

Y

Yoga 173, 175, 179, 218-220

Yogurt 130, 137, 141, 142, 144, 145

Yohimbe 203, 257, 260

NOTES

NOTES

NOTES

NOTES

NOTES

NOTES

NOTES

NOTES

NOTES

NOTES